# CREATING HEALTHY HABITS FOR LIFE

## Part I

## C·R·E·A·T·I·O·N Health

### LIFE GUIDE #1

*For Individual Study and Small Group Use*

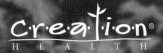

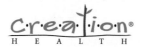

CREATION Health Life Guide #1
Copyright © MMXII by Florida Hospital
Published by Florida Hospital Publishing
900 Winderley Place, Suite 1600
Maitland, Florida 32751

To Extend *the* Health *and* Healing Ministry *of* Christ

| | |
|---|---|
| PUBLISHER AND EDITOR-IN-CHIEF: | Todd Chobotar |
| MANAGING EDITOR: | David Biebel, DMin |
| PRODUCTION: | Lillian Boyd |
| PROMOTION: | Laurel Dominesey |
| COPY EDITOR: | Mollie Braga |
| PHOTOGRAPHER: | Timothy Brown |
| DESIGN: | Carter Design, Inc. |
| PEER REVIEWERS: | Bradford Eakins, MDiv; Robert Hayes |
| | Gerald Wasmer, MDiv; Greg Ellis, MDiv |
| | Mary Lou Caskey; Sabine Vatel, DMin |
| | Andy McDonald, DMin; Tim Goff, MDiv |
| | Rick Szilagyi, DMin; James Dill, MD |
| | Andre VanHeerden; Paul Campoli, MDiv |
| | Jeff Cinquemani, MA; Eric Doran, DMin |

For volume discounts please contact special sales at:
HealthProducts@FLHosp.org | 407-303-1929

*Cataloging-in-Publication Data for this book*
*is available from the Library of Congress.*
*Printed in the United States of America.*
PR 14 13 12 11 10 9 8 7 6 5 4 3 2 1
ISBN: 978-0-9839881-1-3

For more life-changing resources visit:
**FloridaHospitalPublishing.com**
**Healthy100Churches.org**
**CREATIONHealth.com**
**Healthy100.org**

# CONTENTS

Introduction – Welcome to CREATION Health     4

1. Life Beyond the Crib     6

2. Banana Life     16

3. Making Happiness Happen     28

4. Cruising     42

5. What are Habits?     54

6. It's All About Movement     66

7. Defining Your New Habit     78

8. Small Steps are a Big Deal     90

About the Author     101

Notes     102

Resources     105

**DOWNLOAD YOUR FREE LEADER RESOURCE**

Are you a small group leader? We've created a special resource to help you lead an effective CREATION Health discussion group. Download at: **CREATIONHealth.com/LeaderResources**

# WELCOME TO CREATION HEALTH

Congratulations on your choice to use this resource to improve your life! Whether you are new to the concept of CREATION Health or are a seasoned expert, this book was created for you. CREATION Health is a faith-based health and wellness program based on the Bible's Creation story. This book is part of a Life Guide series seeking to help you apply eight elegantly simple principles for living life to the full.

The letters of the CREATION acronym stand for:

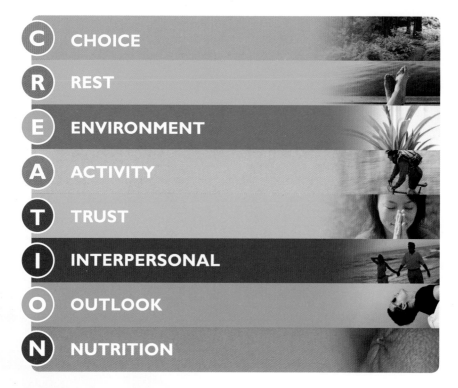

**C** CHOICE

**R** REST

**E** ENVIRONMENT

**A** ACTIVITY

**T** TRUST

**I** INTERPERSONAL

**O** OUTLOOK

**N** NUTRITION

In John 10:10 Jesus said, "I have come that they may have life, and have it to the full" (NIV). The Greek word used for life is "zoe," which means the absolute fullness of life…genuine life…a life that is active, satisfying, and filled with joy.

That is why CREATION Health takes a life-transforming approach to total person wellness – mentally, physically, spiritually and socially – with the eight universal principles of health. Where did these principles come from?

The book of Genesis describes how God created the earth and made a special garden called Eden as a home for his first two children, Adam and Eve. One of the first and finest gifts given to them was abundant health. By examining the Creation story we can learn much about feeling fit and living long, fulfilling lives today.

As you begin this journey toward an improved lifestyle, remember that full health is more than the absence of disease and its symptoms. It's a realization that God desires each of his children – people like you and me whom he loves and cares about – to have the best that this life can offer. It is trusting that your Creator has a plan for your life.

Is there any good parent who doesn't want the best for their child? No. So it makes sense that God would want his best for us. Naturally, human freedom of choice sometimes makes life messy, so not everything can or will be perfect as it once was. But that doesn't mean we shouldn't take a good look at the earliest records of humans found in the Bible to see if there is something special that can be gleaned.

This book – and the other seven in the Life Guide series – takes a deep dive into CREATION Health and translates the fundamental concepts into easy-to-follow steps. These guides include many questions designed to help you or your small group plumb the depths of every principle and learn strategies for integrating the things you learn into everyday life. As a result, you will discover that embracing the CREATION Health prescription can help restore health, happiness, balance, and joy to life.

The CREATION Health Lifestyle has a long, proven history of wellness and longevity – worldwide! People just like you are making a few simple changes in their lives and living longer, fuller lives. They are getting healthy, staying healthy, and are able to do the things they love, well into their later years. Now is the time to join them by transforming your habits into a healthy lifestyle.

If you would like to learn more about the many resources available, visit **CREATIONHealth.com**. If you would like to learn more about how to live to a Healthy 100, visit **Healthy100.org** or visit **Healthy100Churches.org**.

Welcome to CREATION Health,

**Todd Chobotar**
*Publisher and Editor-in-Chief*

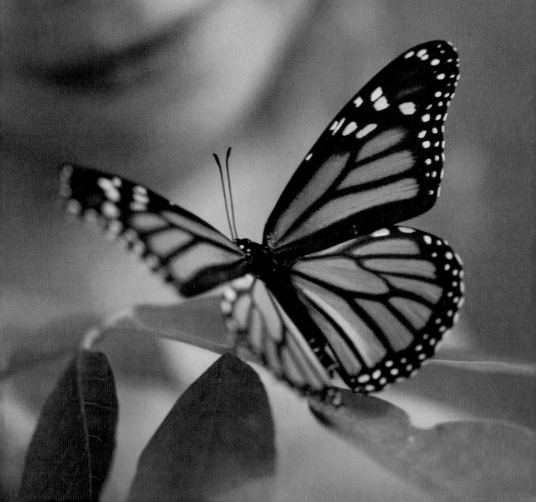

# LIFE BEYOND THE CRIB

*LESSON ONE*

# WARM UP

Choose one or both questions to discuss (if in group setting) or write out your answers on a separate sheet (for individual use):

**1.  What is your idea of *fun*?**[1]

...................................................................................
...................................................................................
...................................................................................
...................................................................................
...................................................................................
...................................................................................
...................................................................................

**2.  As a child, what did you want to be when you grew up?**[2]

...................................................................................
...................................................................................
...................................................................................
...................................................................................
...................................................................................
...................................................................................
...................................................................................

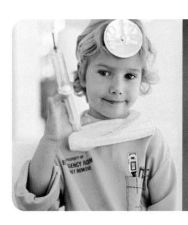

> *"The greatest danger for most of us is not that our aim is too high and we miss it, but that it is too low and we reach it."*
>
> **MICHELANGELO**

# DISCOVERY

Imagine four-month-old, sandy-haired David playing contently in his 3' by 3' crib. He sits upright dressed in a blue, one-piece jumper outfit from Grammy. The baby bangs randomly on the multi-colored buttons sticking up from a raised plastic platform. When one button goes down, another pops up. Giggling with each whack, he suddenly burps up breakfast that dribbles down his chin.

Due to his mother's extreme concern over potential injuries and illness, David is rarely taken outside the house and spends most of his waking hours crawling around the ever-present crib. For his one year birthday, his parents purchase a larger, taller, 5' by 5' enclosure. Mom is pleased that no harm has befallen her beloved boy during his inaugural twelve months.

Five years later, the crib is upgraded to a spacious 8' by 8.' In consultation with David, it is decided that he will get his elementary school education within its familiar, softly webbed walls. Years later, friends and relatives are invited to his eighth grade graduation where he marches around the crib in a black cap and gown while a pre-recorded processional plays brightly in the background. Tears of joy and satisfaction course down his mother's cheeks as she thinks to herself, "All these years and not one accident. No classroom interaction or sports, but no injuries or serious diseases either."

Eventually David's living quarters is expanded to become a network of five cribs with custom-built walkways as connectors. He thoroughly enjoys the larger space and is able to eventually take all of his high school and college courses in there by correspondence. Exactly six months after receiving his BS in Philosophy, David begins dating a young lady over the Internet. On November 29th of that year they are married in the crib, which is quickly expanded yet again into the nearby porch area.

"That's ridiculous," you'd say, and you would certainly be correct. David did get a college degree, but no one would voluntarily endure such limited choices and experiences. More than anything else it was an opportunity lost. An opportunity lost for multi-faceted personal enrichment, deeper happiness, far greater fulfillment, with expanded opportunities and relationships.

Although not taken to such extremes, the "play it safe" theme that marked David's cocooned, fictional existence can all too easily infect our own psyches to one degree or another. And to the extent that it does, it is an opportunity lost for us as well.

Life can become all too routine and automatic, where we wind up coasting, merely reacting, maneuvering only within the familiar, taking life simply as it comes. We know that there are flat spots in our lives, hiccups, downsides, unfulfilled yearnings and proddings, but it is all too easy to glide. We stagnate and settle in for the long haul.

By way of contrast, according to Scripture, we were created by God to stretch and to grow. Jesus put it this way, "I am come that they may have life, and that they may have it *more abundantly*" (John 10:10, NKJV, emphasis added). Abundant living does not guarantee financial success or freedom from pain and perplexity. It is, however, an invitation to reach higher and live life to the fullest in partnership with the Savior. Abundant living calls us out of our comfort zones, out of the default pathways we have developed over time.

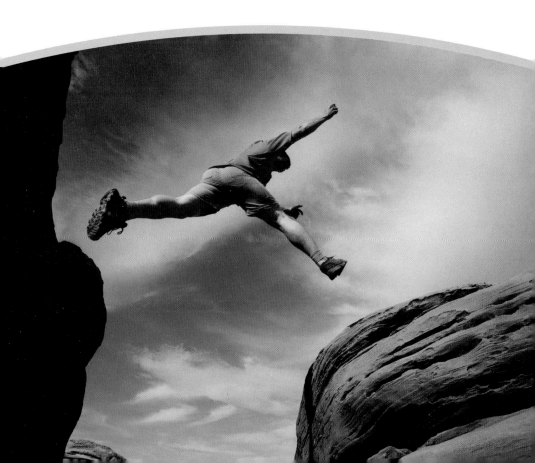

*A man I'll call John recently felt Jesus' call to a fuller life stir again within him. Despite being well over seventy years old, he decided to go for his General Education Development exam, the well-known GED. It is a five-part exam that includes reading, writing, math, science, and social studies, involving seven hours of testing over two or three days. Passing provides a certificate that is considered the equivalent of a high school diploma.*

*Many years before, at age fourteen, John had been forced to drop out of school during eighth grade. At home one night, he failed to correctly spell a word that his father asked about. As a result his dad beat him severely and yelled, "You're so stupid there's no sense sending you back to school anymore. You'll never amount to anything!"*

*John went on to get a job, raise a family, and provide for them faithfully. Now in retirement, he finally chose to fulfill a dream deferred. Much too late in life for a GED to get him a job promotion or any financial gain, John made the extra-ordinary effort simply because he chose to follow Jesus' invitation to stretch and to grow.*

Whether we are nine or ninety, John's example demonstrates well that there need be no hiatus from attaining new heights of satisfaction and joy.

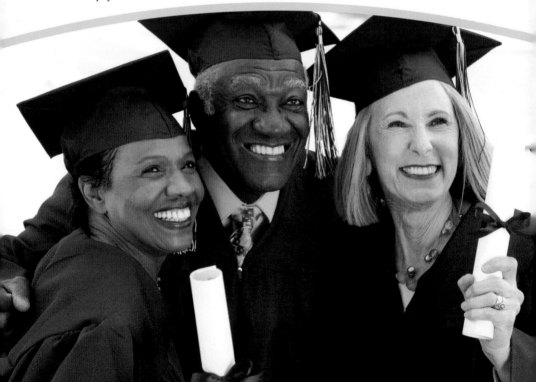

Personal growth in mind, body, and spirit is a major theme in Scripture. For example:

> *"That we henceforth be no more children…*
> *But speaking the truth in love, may grow up into*
> *him in all things, which is the head, even Christ."*
> **EPHESIANS 4:14-15 KJV, EMPHASIS ADDED**
>
> ............................................................
>
> *"I am the vine, ye are the branches: He that*
> *abideth in me, and I in him, the same bringeth*
> *forth much fruit: for without me ye can do nothing."*
> **JOHN 15:5 KJV, EMPHASIS ADDED**
>
> ............................................................
>
> *"Consider the lilies how they grow."*
> **LUKE 12:27 KJV, EMPHASIS ADDED**

God invites us into continual growth for several important reasons:

**1. He loves us and wants the best for us.**
Unlike David's crib loving parents, God's heart is about expansion not constriction, opportunity not limitation, adventure not comfort zones (see 1 Peter 5:7; Ephesians 3:19-21).

**2. Our mind and body are an amazing biological machine,**
built to be challenged and nudged further. As the Scriptures tell us, we are fearfully and wonderfully made (Psalm 139:14). Our entire biological mechanism, with its myriad parts and mind-boggling capabilities, will tend to atrophy if it is allowed to stagnate or function far below its optimal level. We are built for much more than staring at a TV or surviving as a couch potato. We are built for life-long learning, skill building, and progress.

### 3. We are of infinite value to God.

Thinking less of ourselves than God thinks of us narrows our horizons. We discount our own potential, deflect compliments, and keep our grasp well within our reach.

The truth, however, is that we are of great worth in the eyes of God. He looks at us and exclaims loudly so everyone can hear, "Wow! What a wonderful son/daughter!" From God's perspective, we are worth all the health and happiness that life can provide.

Jesus' exalted estimate of our value is not based on who we are but on who he is. It is all about grace and being given what we don't deserve. It is a pure gift from unconditional love. It is his choice to value us to such an extraordinary degree.

As the apostle Peter writes, "It cost God plenty to get you out of that dead-end, empty-headed life you grew up in. He paid with Christ's sacred blood, you know. He died like an unblemished, sacrificial lamb" (1 Peter 1:18-19, MSG).

Heaven's lofty estimate of our worth is not something we can earn or forfeit. It is not based on our good looks, talent, ability, goodness, or the size of our bank account. The source is entirely within the generous heart of our Lord and Friend.

It is as we come to accept God's gracious appraisal that we can learn to say "No" to the inner voices that keep us down and hold us back. We can cast aside any notion that small living is "good enough" and that we should only shop in the marked down bin of life. We can come to believe that God intends us to live life to the fullest.

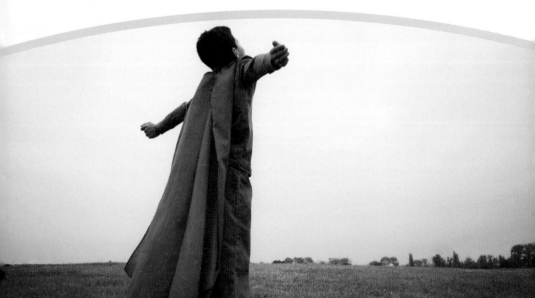

## 4. We are full of talent and potential.

Each of us is a remarkable resource. Besides any other abilities we may have, the apostle Paul teaches in 1 Corinthians 12 that every Christian has received what he calls Spiritual Gifts, special abilities given to us by the Holy Spirit.

The problem comes when we start comparing ourselves to others. Forget that. Concentrate on being who God designed YOU to be. Comparisons are useless because no two people are the same. Don't forego the possibilities God has placed within you just because you can't mirror someone else.

## 5. We are creative people.

"Wait a minute," you might say. "You obviously don't know me very well. I don't have a creative bone in my body." Well, according to Scripture you do! Talking about Jesus, the Bible tells us,

> *"For by Him all things were created that are in heaven and that are on earth, visible and invisible...*
> *All things were created through Him and for Him."*
>
> **COLOSSIANS 1:16, NKJV**

The humble Galilean Carpenter who walked the dusty, rural streets of tiny Nazareth, once created everything that we see and beyond, from flowers to galaxies. Jesus' creative deeds flowed from the abundant *creativity* that constantly surged throughout his being. And when we become his sons and daughters, he puts that creativity within us as well. It may lie dormant or unacknowledged, but it is nonetheless there.

The call to creativity is a gracious invitation to joy and adventure. It is a call to stretch and grow as we strive to reflect the life of the One who brought all things into existence. It is an opportunity to partner with the Spirit who is constantly working to re-create and renew.

Awareness of our God-infused creativity can provide both the impetus and confidence to move beyond any self-imposed limitations of attitude and behavior. It can enable us to step outside the crib and take the initiative to explore new, exciting realms of happiness and abundant living.

Welcome to the new life that lies before you in this series of lessons.

# DISCUSSION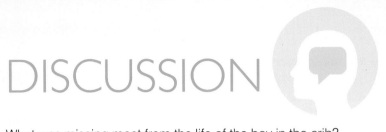

What was missing most from the life of the boy in the crib?

..............................................................................................................................
..............................................................................................................................

What advice would you give to David's mother?

..............................................................................................................................
..............................................................................................................................

What have you done in the last five years that was a stretch for you?

..............................................................................................................................
..............................................................................................................................

Do you feel an inner yearning or prodding to enhance your life in some way? Describe it as best you can.

..............................................................................................................................
..............................................................................................................................

How do you relate to the fact that you are worth an infinite amount to God?

..............................................................................................................................
..............................................................................................................................

What one thing might you do to bring more creativity into your life?

..............................................................................................................................
..............................................................................................................................

Describe a time in your life when you felt like you were experiencing "Abundant Living."

..............................................................................................................................
..............................................................................................................................

# SHARING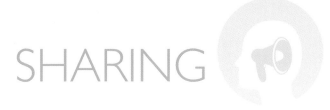

## OPPORTUNITY #1

This section is about an opportunity for you to be a blessing to someone outside of your small group and to also deepen the impact of the lesson on your own life. The group is encouraged to discuss at the end of each meeting what aspects of the lesson they might like to share with someone at home, work, or in the community if the opportunity arises. *There is an "Additional Thought for Sharing" at the end of each lesson as one possibility of something to pass along.*

Start each day asking God to provide opportunities to share and then keep your radar up.

You can be an ambassador and reach people with the good news that Abundant Living is available to all.

### ABUNDANT LIVING THOUGHT

**We can cast aside any notion that small living is "good enough" and that we should only shop in the marked down bin of life. We can come to believe that God intends us to live life to the fullest.**

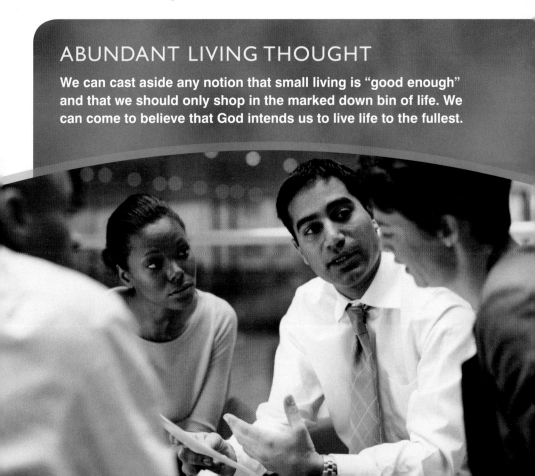

# BANANA LIFE

*LESSON TWO*

# WARM UP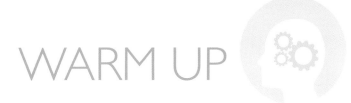

**Feedback: In what ways did God open the door since our last lesson for you to share some part of the lesson with someone else?**

.................................................................................................................................

.................................................................................................................................

.................................................................................................................................

.................................................................................................................................

Choose one or both questions to discuss (if in group setting)
or write out your answers on a separate sheet (for individual use):

1.  **What subject would you choose to write a book about?**[3]

.................................................................................................................................

.................................................................................................................................

.................................................................................................................................

.................................................................................................................................

2.  **What experience or time in your life would you like to re-live? Why?**[4]

.................................................................................................................................

.................................................................................................................................

.................................................................................................................................

.................................................................................................................................

> *"Most people are about
> as happy as they
> make up their minds to be."*
>
> **ABRAHAM LINCOLN**

# DISCOVERY

My wife Ann grew up during the 1950s and '60s in a tiny coastal village on a small island off the coast of Yugoslavia. The only way to the mainland was by boat. She ate well from the family garden and the sea. But bananas were a rare treat due to the exorbitant price-tag. About once a year, she and her younger sister would each be given one banana by their dad.

First they smelled the outside of the unopened, yellow peel from top to bottom, savoring the aroma and mentally anticipating the delicacy so elegantly wrapped inside. Then they slowly pulled away the peel, careful not to injure or break the banana itself. Placing the banana aside, they'd sniff the inside of the peel, several times, pausing between sniffs to bask in its exotic fragrance, trying to lock it into memory long enough to last the many months until the next one came along.

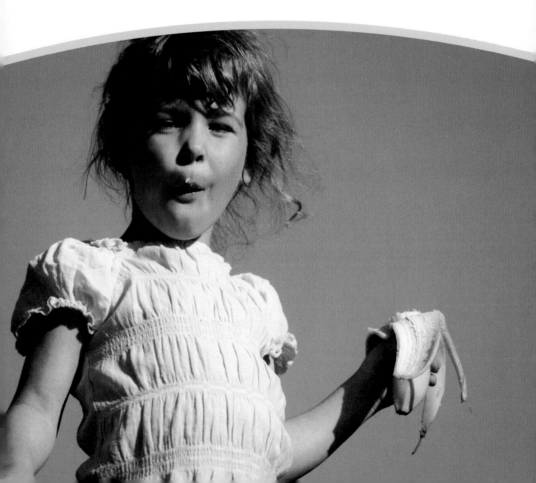

Next, Ann and her sister licked the inside of the peel to get off every bit of banana residue. Then came the finale, the precious, soft, delicate banana itself. Bite by tiny bite, they rolled each piece around inside their mouths until it melted and slipped effortlessly down their throat.

Ann certainly got the most out of what she had available. Nonetheless, at that point she was living a "one banana life." At age sixteen, the family moved to the United States, specifically Queens, NY. That first week Ann and her mom entered a downtown supermarket and there, to their amazement, were *entire bunches* of bananas at an affordable price. She gorged. Such a "many banana life" would never have even occurred to her back on the island.

Many people today are living a "one banana life," not with regard to fruit, but in relation to the level of happiness, satisfaction, and fulfillment they are currently experiencing. They are doing the best they can, but they are living within a constricted framework, a limited awareness of the possibilities. They cannot strive for something they can't envision.

*This lesson and the two that follow will attempt to paint a picture of what it can mean to live an abundant life.* They will point out several important areas for us to consider as we seek to experience a more expansive, fulfilling, enjoyable lifestyle.

When someone wants to build a new home, they don't begin by rushing out and purchasing lumber and flooring and then start sawing and hammering. The first step is to envision what their future home will be like. They peruse magazines, study plans, explore features, inspect construction sites, and talk with friends and experts. First comes the vision, then the "how to's" and materials follow.

Lessons two, three, and four are designed to help you envision not a new house but the new, more fulfilled, happier, healthier life you want to build for yourself. We'll help you form an exciting mental picture by portraying various models, paradigms, and possibilities that you can choose from to construct your own personalized, abundant life. After that, we'll explore the steps you can take in making 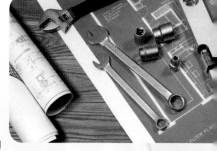 that life a reality. The subjects listed are only a sampling of the many facets of the concept of Abundant Living. They are intended to point the way for your own deeper exploration.

One of the premier models for well-being available today is called "CREATION Health," which was pioneered over the last 100 years by Florida Hospital. Their central focus is "To Extend the Healing Ministry of Christ." The word "CREATION" refers back to the momentous time when God brought life on planet Earth into existence (Genesis 1 & 2). As the Bible record indicates, "Then God looked over all he had made, and he saw that it was very good!" (Genesis 1:31, NLT). *That era holds a unique place in the annals of human history.*

Over the past thousands of years, various civilizations and people groups have arisen, such as:

*Egyptians*
*Greeks*
*Medes*
*Persians*
*Romans*
*Incas*
*Aztecs*
*Chinese*
*Assyrians*
*Sumerian*
*Babylonians, and others.*

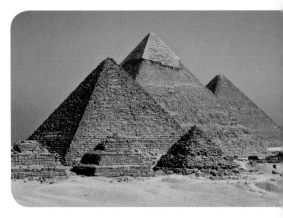

They were characterized by insights into many important areas of life including writing, transportation, art, architecture, systems of government, laws, math, drama, science, pottery, philosophy, agriculture, etc.

But Scripture talks about a period of human history that supersedes them all. It was a special time, unlike any other. It was so unique that it might be compared to traveling to an entirely different planet in some far flung portion of the universe.

It started when God created all of the vegetation, plants, flowers, lakes, oceans, atmosphere, fish, animals, and birds in our world, and finally, Adam and Eve, whose personal, God-designed residence was called Eden, a gorgeous outdoor sanctuary. It ended with the Fall, when man sinned and evil poisoned all. We don't know how long the interval was between Creation and the Fall, but it was an interlude of extraordinary happiness and well-being.

The numerous negative elements that have characterized society down through the ages were completely unknown to Adam and Eve back then. In fact, they weren't even part of the first couple's vocabulary. There was no:

Decay
Cancer
High Blood Pressure
Cardiac Arrest
Diabetes
Death
Divorce
Anger
Depression
Pain
Anxiety
Fear
Insecurity
Smog
Crime
Starvation
War
Recession
Alienation from God

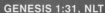

"Then God looked over
all he had made,
and he saw
that it was very good!"

**GENESIS 1:31, NLT**

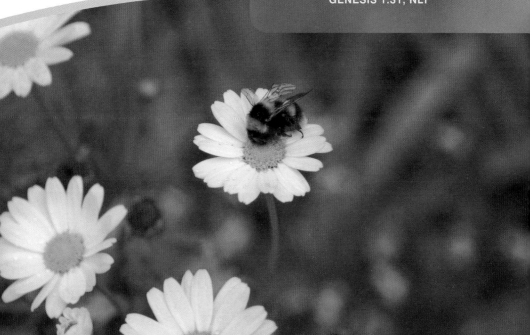

It is from this amazing period of human history before sin that the principles of CREATION Health are derived. We want to recover, as much as possible, the key elements from that dream-like age and bring them forward into today. Normally, going back in time leads to more primitive, ineffective approaches to wellness. In this case, by going all the way back to the beginning, we reach the pinnacle of health. We are able to tap into the ideal, which becomes the basis for abundant living now.

This approach to abundant living uses the word CREATION not only to reference the time of Adam and Eve, but also as an acronym that highlights certain key, life-enhancing principles from that pristine time period. These concepts, listed below, might be considered puzzle pieces that, taken together, portray an image of optimal living.

This paradigm will be explored more fully in subsequent lesson series. At this point, let's simply summarize what each of the letters in the acronym represents.

## CHOICE

God designed our brains with a frontal lobe located just behind our forehead in order to give us the power of choice. It provides us with the ability to live purposefully and manage our destiny. Rather than being completely controlled by outside forces, we can take control of our existence. For the most part, we are the decisions that we make. Without a frontal lobe, our lives would simply be reactive, directionless, pushed and pulled by whatever came our way.

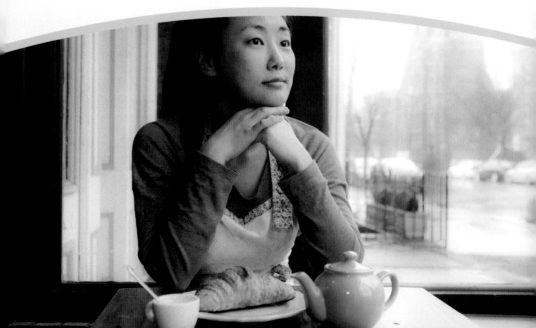

Dogs are like that. I know from experience. My apologies to pet lovers, but I owned three dogs and none of them had a lick of common sense or good judgment. Sure they reacted to stimuli like cats, food, and fire hydrants. But they didn't wake up in the morning and think to themselves, "So what can I do to better myself today?"

I spent big bucks for our completely unruly German Shepherd Husky named Tinker to attend obedience school. As soon as he spied another male canine across the room, he'd go nuts. All his little brain could reason was "dog-male-bad-kill." No sense of time or place. No self-control whatsoever.

I wanted to throw in the towel, but the heavily tattooed, muscle-laden trainer said, "Let me handle him." He put a special collar around Tinker's considerable neck and lifted him up so that the dog's paws barely touched the floor. Tinker didn't utter so much as a peep as he tip-toed around the room like a very furry, novice ballerina.

Thank the Lord I have a functional frontal lobe, or else my wife might have to put a choker on *me*. One of the most crucial elements of abundant living is to understand how to keep our frontal lobe healthy and make wise, life-giving decisions.

## REST

We don't have to wake up in the morning groggy, groping our way to the coffee pot. We don't have to slog through the day and drive home with our head pounding. There is a much better way with invigorating sleep, relaxation breaks during work, refreshing personal activities, and freedom from the corrosive effects of stress.

## ENVIRONMENT

The ideal, serene environment where Adam and Eve lived in Eden has been dramatically altered by today's ever-present noise, clamor, clutter, and endless distractions. God's ideal includes surroundings and inputs that allow us to experience calmness, peace, and renewal.

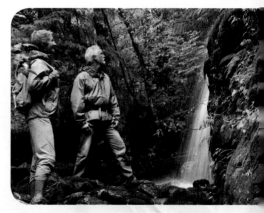

## ACTIVITY

You don't have to be a marathoner or Olympic swimmer to benefit from movement and activity. There are lots of enjoyable ways to get your muscles working, your heart pumping, and your lungs expanding that will add quality to each new day and years to your future. Edward Stanley once observed, "Those who think they have not time for bodily exercise will sooner or later have to find time for illness."[5]

## TRUST IN GOD

Regardless of our current failings, we are all invited to enter into a trust relationship with Jesus. His trustworthiness and unconditional love make him the ideal Partner in our habit change journey. He is the premier path to genuine living:

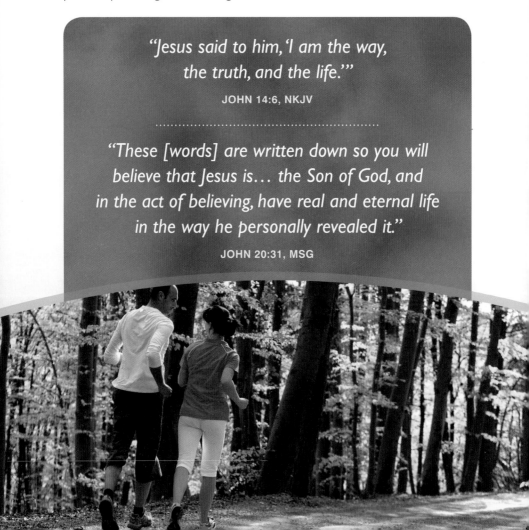

*"Jesus said to him, 'I am the way, the truth, and the life.'"*

**JOHN 14:6, NKJV**

*"These [words] are written down so you will believe that Jesus is… the Son of God, and in the act of believing, have real and eternal life in the way he personally revealed it."*

**JOHN 20:31, MSG**

# INTERPERSONAL RELATIONSHIPS

Close, supportive, caring relationships are an essential part of abundant living. Without them we experience greater anxiety, stress, isolation, depression, and disease. With them we can thrive. As one author put it, "The quality of our relationships, to a large extent, determines the quality of our lives."[6]

# OUTLOOK

The story is told about grandpa's visit to his grandchildren. Every afternoon he would lie down for a nap. One day, as a joke, the grandchildren put Limburger cheese in his mustache. He later awoke, sniffed, and said, "This room stinks." Soon he walked to the kitchen, took a whiff, and determined that it smelled as well. So he walked outside for a breath of fresh air and quickly proclaimed, "The whole world stinks!"[7]

A negative outlook and attitude like that can be toxic to our quality of life. Thankfully, God has provided numerous resources for us to avoid that detour and shift to a much more positive perspective.

# NUTRITION

Fried foods, sugar, and fat can taste terrific. But after they get pro- cessed by our innards and funneled into our blood stream they become robbers and vandals. CREATION Health points us to an alternative, where the foods we eat look fantastic, taste delicious, and make the cells throughout your body shout "Thank you" after every meal.

# CREATION HEALTH

The eight principles listed above, taken together, are often referred to as "Holistic Health" or "Whole Person Health" because they deal with all of the key dimensions of living – physical, mental, spiritual, and social. Each of the eight principles can be integrated into our lives over time in a personalized, systematic, balanced way. To learn more, check out other lessons in the CREATION Health series. You can also refer to: **CREATIONHealth.com** and **Healthy100.org**.

# DISCUSSION
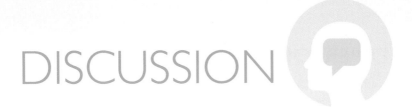

Would you describe yourself as having more of "one banana life" or bunches of bananas? Why?

...................................................................................................

...................................................................................................

If you lived in that pristine time of earth's history prior to sin, what would you be doing today?

...................................................................................................

...................................................................................................

Which of the letters in the CREATION Health acronym captured your interest and/or curiosity the most?

...................................................................................................

...................................................................................................

Tell about a choice you made in the last six months that increased your sense of happiness and well-being?

...................................................................................................

...................................................................................................

How could you put five minute "mini-vacations" in each day in order to enjoy greater rest of mind?

...................................................................................................

...................................................................................................

What small change could you make now to turn your home and/or workplace into more of a haven of calmness and renewal?

...................................................................................................

...................................................................................................

What is one of your favorite Bible verses regarding the trustworthiness of God? Why did you select that verse?

...................................................................................................

...................................................................................................

What would help you become more optimistic?

...................................................................................................

...................................................................................................

What is one of your favorite meals combining great nutrition and taste?

...................................................................................................

...................................................................................................

# SHARING

## OPPORTUNITY #2

- Pray as a group for God to open the way for you to share something from these lessons to help someone else.

- Keep your radar up each day for opportunities.

### ABUNDANT LIVING THOUGHT

**One of the premier models for well-being available today is called CREATION Health – Choice, Rest, Environment, Activity, Trust in God, Interpersonal Relationships, Outlook, and Nutrition.**

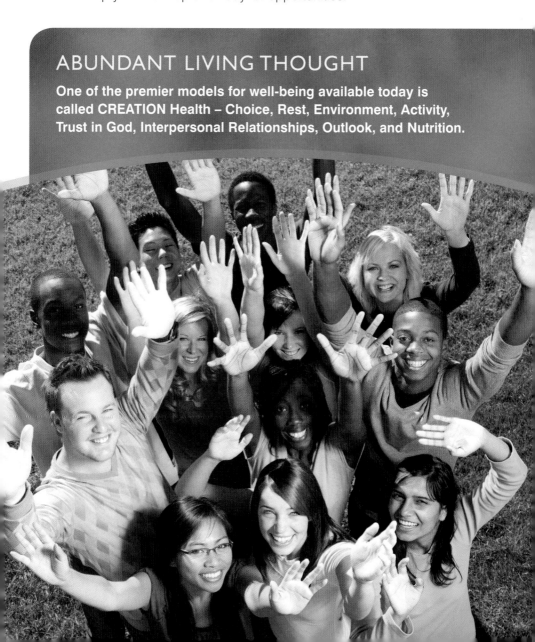

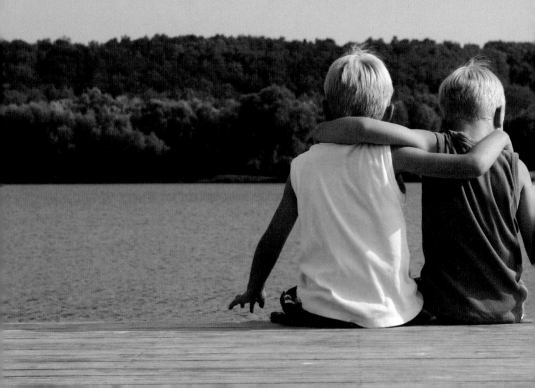

# MAKING
# HAPPINESS HAPPEN

*LESSON THREE*

# WARM UP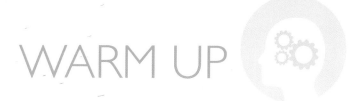

**Feedback: In what ways did God open the door since our last lesson for you to share some part of the lesson with someone else?**

........................................................................................

........................................................................................

........................................................................................

........................................................................................

Choose one or both questions to discuss (if in group setting)
or write out your answers on a separate sheet (for individual use):

1.  **What would cause you to cheer out loud?**[8]

........................................................................................

........................................................................................

........................................................................................

2.  **Where have you traveled in the U.S.? Which place did you like the best and why?**[9]

........................................................................................

........................................................................................

........................................................................................

*"The only legacy greater than the gift of health is the gift of love."*

DR. DES CUMMINGS, JR.

# DISCOVERY

One of the most famous studies regarding twins and the degree to which they experienced abundant living was carried out by researchers at the University of Minnesota. Two participants in the study, identical twins Helen and Audrey from St. Paul, were in their thirties at the time.

During the ten years leading up to the study, Audrey, a graphic designer, had one long-term relationship that went nowhere, eventually married another man, and then moved with him to Chicago.

If the researchers attempted to ascertain Audrey's level of happiness at the time of the study, they wouldn't get an accurate reading from her circumstances. It turns out that the best indicator of Audrey's sense of well-being would be the happiness level of her twin sister Helen. Even if they went back and measured Helen's level of happiness ten years earlier, it would still be very close to what Audrey was experiencing when the "Happiness Twins" study was conducted.

Researchers discovered, to their amazement, that the happiness of one identical twin was a more powerful clue to the other twin's sense of well-being than all the facts and circumstances of their life![10]

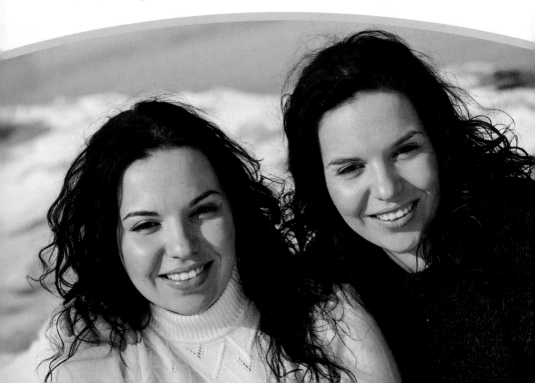

Another study focused on the sense of well-being of identical twins, but this time focused on cases where the twins had been separated in infancy and raised apart. Remarkably, once again they were extremely similar to each other in their happiness scores, even if they grew up in different parts of the country.[11]

But how could that be? Scientists have discovered that *each of us* has what is called a *happiness set point* which is more the result of biology and genetics than anything else. It is a baseline to which we are bound to return, even after significant reverses or dramatic good fortune. Research indicates that our set point cannot be changed and accounts for about 50 percent of our sense of well-being.[12] Identical twins share the same genetic material and have a similar happiness set point.

Studies also reveal that the circumstances of life account for only about 10 percent of our happiness. As hard as it might be to accept, all of the events and life experiences that come our way actually play a relatively minor role, including such things as job, income, housing, marriage, location, and looks. For instance, a well-known study concluded that the wealthiest Americans, who earn more than ten million dollars annually, were only slightly happier than their staff and blue collar employees.[13]

These findings can be represented in the following graphic:[14]

## The Components Of Happiness And A Sense Of Well-Being

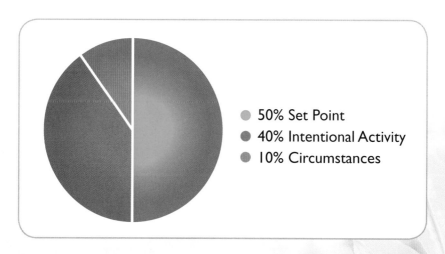

- 50% Set Point
- 40% Intentional Activity
- 10% Circumstances

The great news is that our set point and the circumstances of life are not the final word. We can choose to rise above them. *About 40 percent of our happiness can be determined by our own actions and way of thinking.* We can either be controlled by our genes and life circumstances, or we can proactively build into our lives happiness-producing activities that can permanently raise our sense of well-being if they become an integral part of our attitude and lifestyle. *Our happiness set point might be fixed, but that does not mean our happiness level can't be significantly higher.*[15]

Abundant living is within everyone's grasp, but it won't just happen. It takes commitment and must be intentionality practiced on a regular basis. *Happiness is not something that you find, it is something you create.*

In addition to the CREATION Health principles presented in Lesson 2, this lesson and the next will present more activities that have the potential to boost your overall sense of happiness and well-being. Look them over carefully and find one or two that are a good fit for you and consider the others later. Think of these activities not as a long to-do-list to make you feel guilty but as a cafeteria of opportunities to grow.

Different activities have different impacts on people. It is crucial to discover the ones that work for you. You will tend to maintain abundant living endeavors if they fit your goals, play to your strengths, capture your interest, and don't turn your schedule completely upside down.

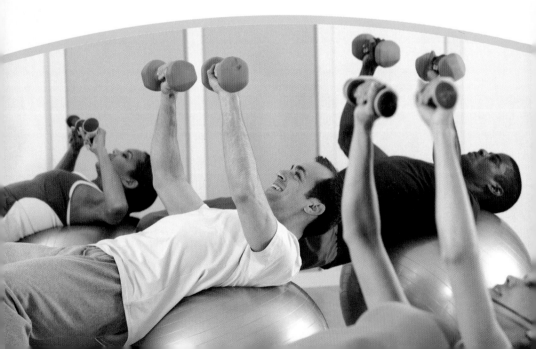

# GRATITUDE

The world's most prominent researcher on the benefits of gratitude, Robert Emmons, defines it as, "A knowing awareness that we are the recipients of goodness. In gratitude we remember the contribution that others have made for the sake of our well-being."[16] It also includes the notion of underserved merit.

Each year a teacher in a psychology class gives her undergraduate students the assignment to write a gratitude letter. One of those students, Nicole, describes her experience in writing to her mom:

> *I felt overwhelmed with a sense of happiness. I noticed I was typing very quickly, probably because it was very easy for me to express gratitude that was long overdue. As I was typing, I could feel my heart beating faster and faster… Towards the end of the letter, as I reread what I had already, I began to get teary eyed and even a little bit choked-up. Expressing my gratitude to my mom overwhelmed me to such a point that tears streamed down my face.*[17]

Later that week, frustrated with her lack of progress on a research paper, Nicole decided to take a break and again read the letter. Instantly a smile broke out and her mood quickly shifted. She felt much happier and less stressed for the rest of the day. Such is the power of gratitude. Consistently practiced, it can be life changing.

Gratitude is a powerful way of acknowledging the presence of God in our life and the numerous gifts he brings our way. It is being thankful for what we have, see, hear, and feel. We need not be thankful for pain and tragedy, but we can help ourselves immensely by being grateful for good things that happen despite them.

Science has now confirmed the many benefits of gratitude. Studies at the Universities of California and Miami concluded that keeping a weekly gratitude journal resulted in people exercising more regularly, having fewer illnesses, feeling better about their lives overall, and being more optimistic. These thankful individuals also made better progress toward their most important goals – academic, interpersonal, or health-based.[18]

Stephen Post, PhD, professor of bioethics at Case Western Reserve University's School of Medicine, has discovered that gratitude increases our body's natural antibodies, helps us focus mentally, avoid depression, and have healthier blood pressure and heart rate.[19]

Researchers have discovered some important guidelines for making gratitude an integral part of your abundant living lifestyle:[20]

1. **It is more impactful to record your blessing once a week than every day. Otherwise it can become routine and simply another part of your to-do list.**

2. **Keep the way you express thankfulness fresh. You may keep a journal for a few weeks, then simply keep track mentally for awhile, or utilize the arts such as painting, or share your thinking with a friend.**

3. **Make thankfulness a regular part of your prayer life.**

4. **Express gratitude directly to people.**

5. **Don't just look for big things. Focus primarily on the small, often overlooked blessings. Life is mostly the small stuff. One author highlights our tendency to overlook what's all around us,**

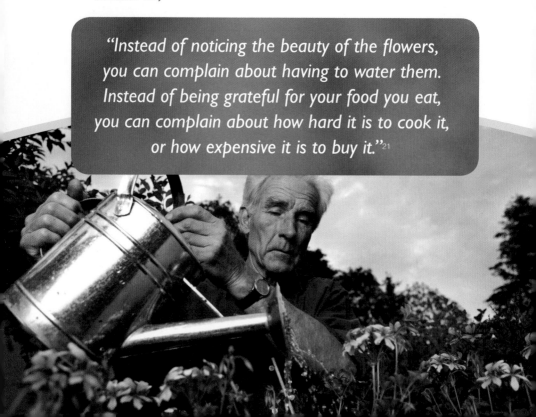

*"Instead of noticing the beauty of the flowers, you can complain about having to water them. Instead of being grateful for your food you eat, you can complain about how hard it is to cook it, or how expensive it is to buy it."*[21]

# ACTS OF KINDNESS AND GENEROSITY

One morning an education consultant was making her rounds of schools, when she noticed something colorful on her car's windshield. As she got closer, she realized that it was a gorgeous yellow rose, diamoned with dew. There was no note attached. Coupled with the morning sunshine, this unexpected gift created a wave of positive feelings and wonderment. The giver would never know about the many times that anonymous rose inspired the consultant to put roses on other people's windshields in joyful response. They had started a chain of kindness that multiplied to uplift many.[22]

All four Gospels record the story of the miraculous feeding of 5,000 men and, most likely, at least twice that number of women and children (Matthew 14:13-21; Mark 6:35-44; Luke 9:10-17; John 6:1-13). Jesus was teaching all day and concern arose that people on the crowded hillside would be getting hungry and it was a long journey home.

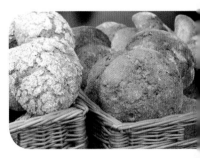

The primary focus is on Christ who multiplied five loaves and two fishes to feed the masses with twelve baskets left over. We should also reflect on the little boy who offered his few morsels in the first place – "Hey mister, you can have my lunch." Undoubtedly his mother had packed the lunch before he left home to listen to the Master. The lad had become so engrossed in Jesus' teaching that he'd forgotten to eat. Everyone else had apparently already downed their own provisions long ago. The youngster generously offered his meal even though it was late in the day and his own stomach must have been growling big time.[23]

The five loaves were only little barley buns, the food of the poor. The fish were nothing more than sardines, used as a kind of relish.[24] Someone sitting next to him might have elbowed him and counseled, "Might as well eat that yourself, boy, it isn't going to make a lick of difference in this crowd." Despite the apparent futility of the gesture, the youngster gave what he could and Jesus provided the miracle of multiplication. The same can happen in our own lives. As we partner with God, he takes our little acts of kindness and generosity and multiplies them to bless others.

Just like the little boy must have gone home with renewed delight and satisfaction at what his gift had become, helping others reverberates to bless and uplift our own lives. Dave Toycen states, "Generous acts have the unique ability to lift us to a higher level where we are more human, more the person we really want to be."[25] So what's in your lunch bag?

Volunteering is one of the most widespread and rewarding ways to spread kindness and generosity. Researchers have discovered tremendous reflex benefits for the giver. In his book, *The Healing Power of Doing Good*, Allan Luks surveyed 3,000 volunteers serving twenty organizations and concluded that service helped sustain good health and reduce the impact of diseases, both physical and psychological.[26]

As the Scriptures indicate, "A generous man will himself be blessed, for he shares his food with the poor" (Proverbs 22:9, NIV).

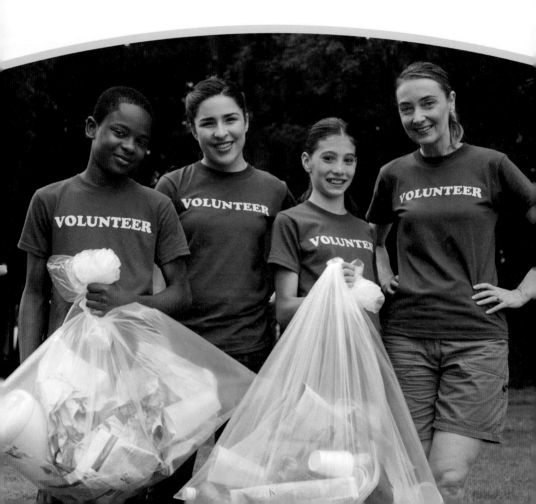

# SAVOR LIFE'S JOYS

Savoring is like sucking up the last bit of a milkshake with the noisy, prolonged "sssllllrrrppp" of a straw. It's like catching a whiff of sweet floral scent on a walk and taking time to seek out the source. It's like replaying a favorite tune over and over to let every note have its day.

Research indicates that savorers are more self-confident, outgoing, more hopeful, less neurotic, and less likely to experience depression, stress, or guilt.[27] Here are some pointers to enhance your savory experience:[28]

1. **Be present in the present.**

2. **Relish everyday experiences.**

3. **Reminisce and reflect with family and friends.**

4. **Recall happy days.**

5. **Celebrate upbeat news.**

6. **Be aware of beauty.**

7. **Take pleasure in what your senses absorb.**

# INCREASE FLOW EXPERIENCES

A "Flow Experience" is when you get so absorbed in something captivating and enjoyable that you lose track of time. Time just seems to flow quickly by. To boost your happiness level, build more of these types of experiences into your life. Flow experiences happen most often when we are pursuing activities we care deeply about.[29]

> *"A generous man will himself be blessed,*
> *for he shares his food with the poor."*
>
> **PROVERBS 22:9, NIV**

# ACT HAPPY

Many times our feelings follow our actions. In a study, one group of students were told to hold a felt-tip marker in their teeth, mimicking a smile, and the other group held a marker between puckered lips, mimicking a frown. The two groups were then shown cartoons and the first group actually found them to be considerably funnier.[30] This study and others like it indicate that choosing to adopt facial expressions and characteristics of happiness can go a long way to helping you experience inner joy.

# FORGIVE YOURSELF AND OTHERS

The subject of forgiveness is both crucial and difficult. It deserves much more exploration than can be devoted to it here.* Nonetheless, abundant living can remain at arm's length if we cling to either guilt over our shortcomings of the past or bitterness over the awful way we were treated by someone else.

Anyone suffering from self-punishment over mistakes of the past can take comfort in God's amazing grace. The apostle John wrote, "If we confess our sins, He is faithful and just to forgive us our sins and to cleanse us from all unrighteousness" (1 John 1:9, NKJV).

And refusing to forgive others for past wrongs is like taking poison ourselves in order to get back at someone else. Forgiveness is not forgetting or condoning. It is not about the perpetrator. It is about releasing us from the hate that stifles our joy.

In order to insulate ourselves from the corrosive effects of prolonged anger, forgiveness should become a habitual attitude and way of life.

As you reflect on the various paths to happiness presented in this lesson, choose to enter a journey of discovery to determine which ones you are willing to make happen in your own life.

*For further guidance on forgiveness, see the book Forgive to Live, by Dr. Dick Tibbits

# NOTES:

........................................................

........................................................

........................................................

........................................................

........................................................

........................................................

........................................................

........................................................

........................................................

........................................................

........................................................

........................................................

........................................................

........................................................

........................................................

........................................................

........................................................

*"If we confess our sins,
He is faithful
and just to forgive
us our sins and to
cleanse us from
all unrighteousness."*

1 JOHN 1:9, NKJV

# DISCUSSION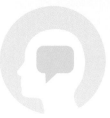

How did you react to the percentages in the graph on page 31?

..............................................................................................................................

..............................................................................................................................

Were you surprised that life circumstances, on average, make up only 10 percent of our happiness? Why?

..............................................................................................................................

..............................................................................................................................

Do you feel that winning one million dollars would make you permanently happier? Why or why not?

..............................................................................................................................

..............................................................................................................................

Has there been a time when you expressed gratitude and were personally uplifted as a result, like Nicole?

..............................................................................................................................

..............................................................................................................................

How beneficial do you think it would be for you to keep a "Gratitude Journal"? What could you be grateful for from the previous week?

..............................................................................................................................

..............................................................................................................................

Why do you think Jesus chose to use the little boy's lunch when he could have created plenty of food from nothing?

..............................................................................................................................

..............................................................................................................................

What is a positive experience you have had in the past as a volunteer? How did it benefit you?

..............................................................................................................................

..............................................................................................................................

Which of the items on the list under "Savor Life's Joys" would you be most likely use?

..............................................................................................................................

..............................................................................................................................

Does the suggestion to "Act Happy" seem workable to you? Why?

..............................................................................................................................

..............................................................................................................................

# SHARING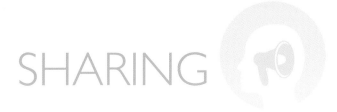

## OPPORTUNITY #3:

- Pray as a group for God to open the way for you to share something from these lessons to help someone else.

- Keep your radar up each day for opportunities.

## ABUNDANT LIVING THOUGHT

**About 40 percent of our happiness can be determined by our own actions and way of thinking.**

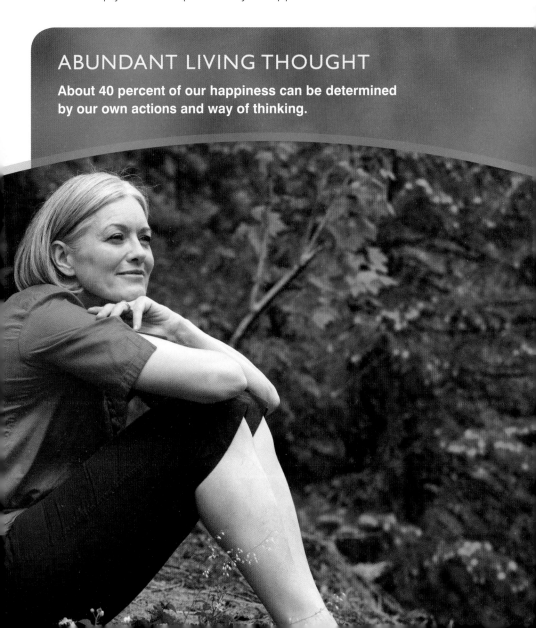

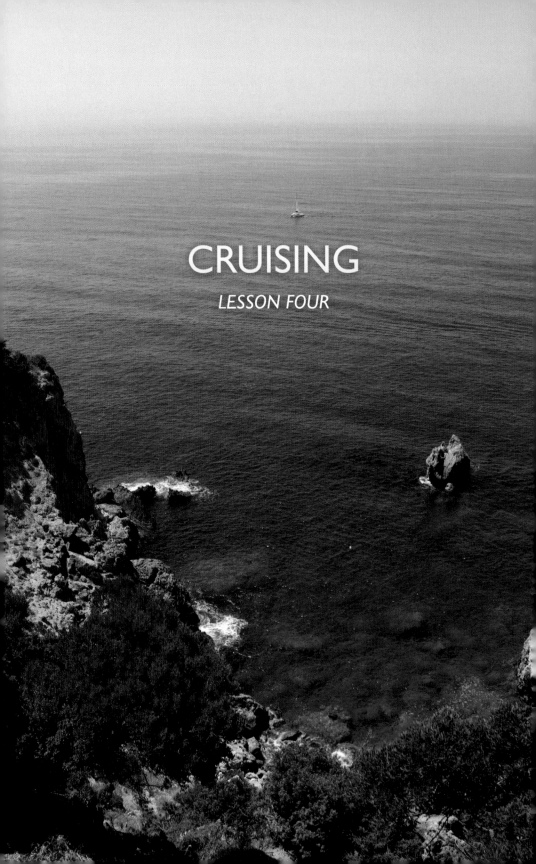

# CRUISING

*LESSON FOUR*

# WARM UP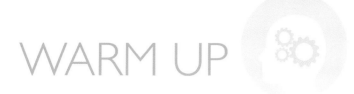

**Feedback: In what ways did God open the door since our last lesson for you to share some part of the lesson with someone else?**

..................................................................................
..................................................................................
..................................................................................
..................................................................................

Choose one or both questions to discuss (if in group setting)
or write out your answers on a separate sheet (for individual use):

1.  **Who is a person you most admire, past or present? Why?**[31]

..................................................................................
..................................................................................
..................................................................................

2.  **What's been one of the most helpful pieces of advice you've ever received?**

..................................................................................
..................................................................................
..................................................................................

> *"God longs to lead you, to show you hope and a positive vision of your future."*
>
> **HEATHER NEAL**

# DISCOVERY

I stared in wonderment as dad backed the long trailer and its hulking cargo down the dirt driveway by our home. Atop the trailer sat a 21' cabin cruiser in a state of considerable disrepair. The boat had obviously seen much better days. Planks were conspicuously missing from the bottom and sides; windows were smashed; no motor, drive shaft or propeller; holes in the decking; seats torn out; no navigation lights or steering wheel; paint peeling everywhere; and dry rot in too many places.

"Isn't she a beauty!" dad exclaimed.

"Uh, yah, I guess so," I replied. "But it's a little beat up isn't it?"

"Don't worry about that, son," he said, "I have a plan."

I was skeptical but knew that once a dream took root deep within dad's brain it would somehow be carried out as fully as time and finances would allow.

One night dad brought home another treasure – a Chevy V-8 car motor he planned to use in the boat. He got it for peanuts because it had, as he explained, "seized up," which meant it had been sitting outside for so long that everything inside was immobilized by rust. Perched on a cement wall, it eventually yielded to gallons of de-ruster and intricate mechanical surgery.

On a Sunday afternoon, my father attached the reclaimed motor to a battery, poured some semi-explosive mixture down the carburetor, and cranked it up. "Bang, bang, rattle, pow." The V-8 came to life belching white smoke. I scrambled up the embankment and hid, trembling, behind a large oak. Dad dashed behind a nearby stand of bushes. Soon the semi-explosive mixture was used up and the thing sputtered to a noisy stop.

Characteristically, dad came out from the shrubbery shouting, "Fantastic! Absolutely fantastic," as he saw another piece of his outsized dream come alive.

Elderly neighbors who had accumulated various boat parts in their basements showed up, parts in tow, offering them in exchange for a future ride on the high seas. The cabin cruiser eventually took shape and was launched with great ceremony. For years afterward we delighted in its ability to add to our otherwise limited adventure.

God is a dreamer who embraces wrecks as well. He declared through the prophet Jeremiah,

"'For I know the plans I have for you,' declares the LORD, 'plans to prosper you and not to harm you, plans to give you hope and a future'" (Jeremiah 29:11, NIV).

God has his own plans for each of our lives. No matter what shape we are currently in, he looks at us and declares, "Fantastic, beautiful," because he has a vision of a life that can be ours. He has the expertise and resources to make it happen if we are only willing.

At the heart of God's vision is for us to "prosper." Although it includes financial stability, he is not talking about us becoming millionaires. The broader definition of prosper includes all the various elements of an abundant life.[32] That vision is reiterated through the apostle John, in the New Testament,

"Beloved, I pray that you may prosper in all things and be in health, just as your soul prospers" (3 John 2, NKJV).

In this lesson, we explore more elements of God's abundant living vision. As you compare your current life to what's available, you can hopefully conclude, "I know that I would feel happier and have a greater sense of well-being if I adopted these particular practices and ways of thinking and, by God's grace, incorporated them into my lifestyle over time."

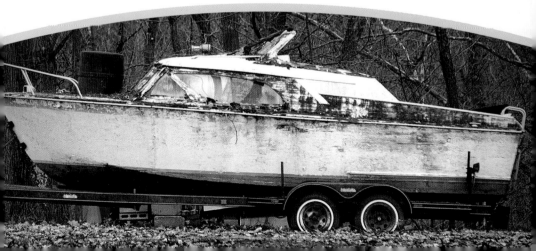

# HUMOR

Small children typically laugh about four hundred times each day, but adults only about seventeen.[33] We would do well to heed what the Scriptures told us centuries ago, "A cheerful heart is good medicine, but a broken spirit saps a person's strength" (Proverbs 17:22, NLT).

Science has now confirmed the truth of those words. Francisco Contreras, MD and surgical oncologist, writes, "One bout of anger will diminish the efficiency of your immune system for six hours, but one good laugh will increase the efficiency of your immune system for twenty-four hours."[34]

"The old saying that 'laughter is the best medicine,' definitely appears to be true when it comes to protecting your heart," says Michael Miller, MD, director of the Center for Preventive Cardiology at the University of Maryland Medical Center.[35] Laughter reduces stress, deepens social and family bonds, lowers blood pressure, and increases tolerance for pain.[36]

Because of humor's benefits, it is also important to give *recreation and play* an important place among our priorities. It is not a luxury to only engage in if time permits, but an essential part of any happiness strategy. Irish playwright George Bernard Shaw said: "We don't stop playing because we grow old; we grow old because we stop playing."[37]

Julia Cameron suggests that we make an appointment with ourselves to take two hours a week to do something creative and/or fun even though we erroneously tell ourselves that we don't have time.[38]

And don't forget to laugh at yourself. Not taking ourselves quite so seriously is another great opportunity for a good hearty chuckle.

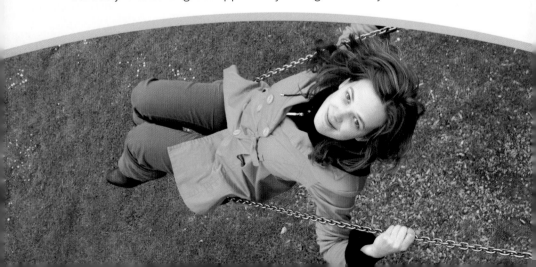

# MONITOR YOUR ENERGY LEVEL

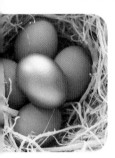 You're probably familiar with the fable of the goose that laid the golden egg. A farmer takes a strange looking, yellow colored egg from one of the geese to be appraised and is told that it is pure gold. Day after day he sells the eggs and becomes fabulously wealthy. Eventually he gets greedy, can't wait for the funds, and decides to kill the goose to get all of the eggs at once. However, when he opens the goose there is no gold. He has destroyed the source that produced them.

In life, our tendency is to measure our effectiveness by how much we *produce* [the eggs]. But unless we pay equal attention to the *capacity to produce* [the goose], we will be shortsighted and become depleted. Abundant living depends on striking the balance between production and production capacity, or P and PC.[39]

The keys are to (1) equally value *both* P and PC, and (2) monitor our energy level on a regular basis. Taking time for rejuvenation and self-care is not a sign of weakness. Nor is it something we should feel guilty about. It is fundamental and essential. Different people have different energy requirements and we each need to find our own way.

When I arrived to give my first seminar at a large spiritual convention, I was picked up at the airport and placed in a van with another presenter who appeared to be hyper. He immediately dominated the conversation indicating how pleased he was that people could hear his material and have a chance to learn about his "powerful" books, articles, CDs, DVDs, etc. As his entrepreneurial spirit oozed all over the interior, I began to wonder if he also ran a worldwide chain of religious restaurants and spas.

After my initial presentation I hung around the meeting area trying to emulate speakers like my van partner, engaging strangers, wandering from group to group chatting. By the end of the day I was so utterly drained that I could barely drag myself back to the motel.

I shared the experience with my counselor, and I'll never forget his advice. "Don't compare yourself with anyone. You're more introverted and need rest. Balance your outflow of energy with the inflow. My advice is to give your talk, shake a few hands, then hurry back to the motel for the remainder of the day to recoup." I've tried to implement that P/PC principle in all the years since.

Another aspect of energy flow is to think of it in the context of giving and receiving. In many ways you get what you give. If you want love, learn to love those around you. If you want respect, offer it to others. If you want joy, choose to give it away first. As one author puts it:

> *"Learn to be a giver of all that you desire, and then graciously receive the gifts that will begin to flow naturally into your own life."*[40]

We don't give in order to receive. But we cannot expect to receive unless we are first of all willing to share.

# BALANCE GROWTH IN ALL FOUR AREAS OF LIFE

Another way to address the need for balance in our lives is to look at the fourfold areas of spiritual, mental, physical, and social. Christ gave us a compelling example as highlighted by the gospel writer Luke, "Jesus grew in wisdom [mental] and in stature [physical] and in favor with God [spiritual] and all the people [social]" (Luke 2:52, NLT).

These pillars of a happy life are represented in the following graphic:

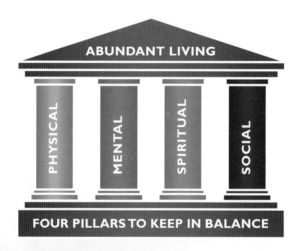

It is important to periodically take stock and see if we have inadvertently been giving attention to some areas at the expense of others. Clear indicators of an imbalance are things like increased stress, anxiety, fatigue, irritability, a lack of sleep, breakdown in relationships, loss of focus, and a feeling of being overwhelmed. Future lessons will examine each of these four pillars further.

# OPTIMIZE YOUR ROLES

The following graphic lists a number of potential roles we have in life. Each role is associated with a line that goes from zero at the center to 10 at the perimeter. A 10 means that you feel that things are going *optimally well for that particular responsibility*. A zero means it is the pits. The goal is to periodically consult this graphic (or one of your own devising) and score yourself for each relevant area by putting a dot on the line where you feel you are at the moment.

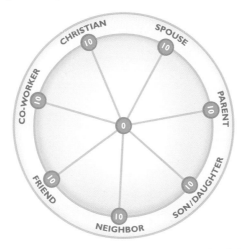

Next, connect all the dots. The graphic below on the left shows a scattered outcome. The one on the right shows a more symmetrical result, which is what you ultimately want in order to move closer to the abundant life God longs for you to have.

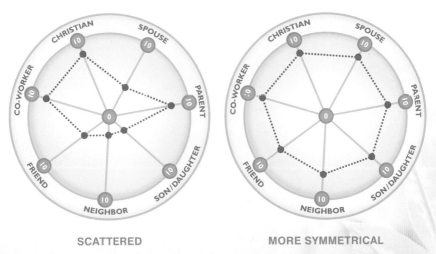

SCATTERED                    MORE SYMMETRICAL

Remember, where you put the dot is not an indicator of time spent but simply your assessment of how well you feel you are fulfilling that particular role. The goal is not equal time, but a greater symmetry of effectiveness. If done periodically, it should reveal some lower scores that need attention and other areas where you have made significant progress.[41] Don't get discouraged and don't try to work on too many roles at once. Pick one or two roles and set some small, realistic, goals for improvement. Then, after progress is made, move on to others. It is an accumulation of tiny steps, over time, that will get you there.

> "A cheerful heart is good medicine, but a broken spirit saps a person's strength."
>
> **PROVERBS 17:22, NLT**

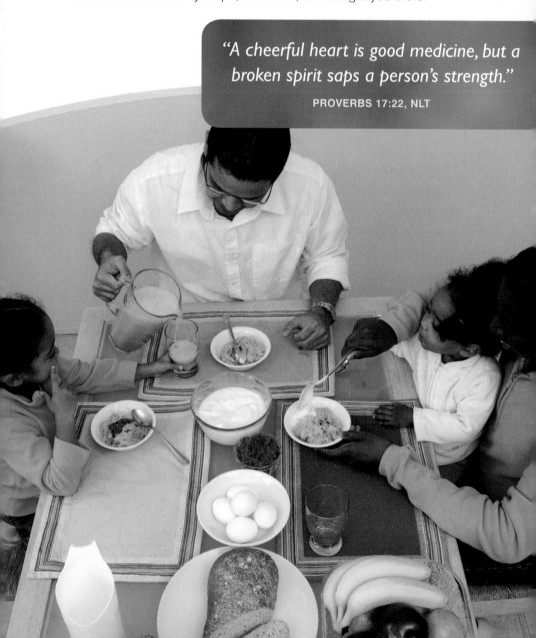

# THE POWER OF FAMILY MEALS

Don't assume that proximity equals meaningful conversation. People can know each other and even live under the same roof for years and never really talk about anything more meaningful than the grocery list or the latest TV program. We need to get outside our own heads and interact with others at more than a surface level in order to feel complete. We need other people's insights and feedback.

Meaningful conversation is often the exception rather than the rule in today's society. One prominent victim is *family dinner*. What used to be taken for granted – gathering several nights a week as a family around the supper table – has been in serious decline. Much more than good nutrition was lost. We also lost the fruits of great conversation – closeness, sharing, affirmation, problem solving, and history sharing.

Numerous studies now make it abundantly clear that the impact of family dinners is way out of proportion to the rather un-dramatic nature of the event itself. *The big key is what occurs during meals – the conversation, modeling, and planned activities*. One of the best sources for dinner activities can be found online at "Families With Purpose," www.familieswithpurpose.com/family-dinner-games.html

Research has also discovered that gathering everyone together for an unhurried meal on a regular basis has the potential to yield tremendous benefits for children.

To find out more, check out the following resources:

**Books:**
- *Drawing Families Together One Meal at a Time* by Jill Kimball
- *The Surprising Power of Family Meals: How Eating Together Makes Us Smarter, Stronger, Healthier and Happier* by Miriam Weinstein
- *The Family Dinner* by Laurie David
- *The Intentional Family* by William J. Doherty

**Websites:**
- *Family Table Time*  www.FamilyTableTime.com
- *Time at The Table*  www.TimeAtTheTable.org
- *Power of Family Meals*  www.PowerOfFamilyMeals.com
- *Casa Family Day*  www.CasaFamilyDay.org
- *Eat Dinner*  www.EatDinner.org

# DISCUSSION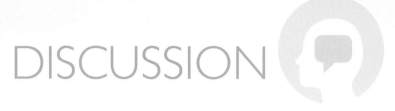

Have you ever turned something that was a wreck into something useful?

........................................................................................................

........................................................................................................

What two or three words could you imagine being part of God's plan for you to prosper?

........................................................................................................

........................................................................................................

What experience did you have lately where you had to laugh at yourself?

........................................................................................................

........................................................................................................

How is your energy balance at present? What could improve that?

........................................................................................................

........................................................................................................

What area of your life – physical, mental, spiritual, or social – is most in need of attention? How could that happen?

........................................................................................................

........................................................................................................

What role are you performing the best in right now and which one is the lowest? How could the lower one be improved? (see the chart "Optimize Your Roles" in this lesson)

........................................................................................................

........................................................................................................

How would you describe a "meaningful conversation"? When was the last time you engaged in one?

........................................................................................................

........................................................................................................

Which of the abundant living suggestions in Lessons 2-4 captures your interest at this point as a potential new habit?

........................................................................................................

........................................................................................................

........................................................................................................

# SHARING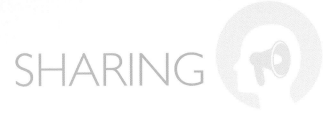

## OPPORTUNITY #4:

- Pray as a group for God to open the way for you to share something from these lessons to help someone else.

- Keep your radar up each day for opportunities.

## ABUNDANT LIVING THOUGHT

Small children typically laugh about four hundred times each day, but adults only about seventeen. We would do well to heed what the Scriptures told us centuries ago, "A cheerful heart is good medicine, but a broken spirit saps a person's strength" Proverbs 17:22, NLT.

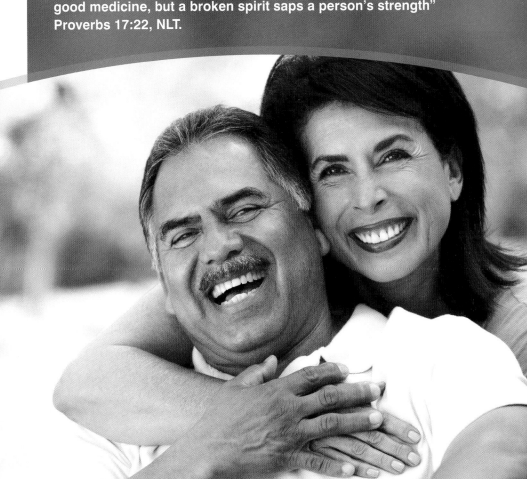

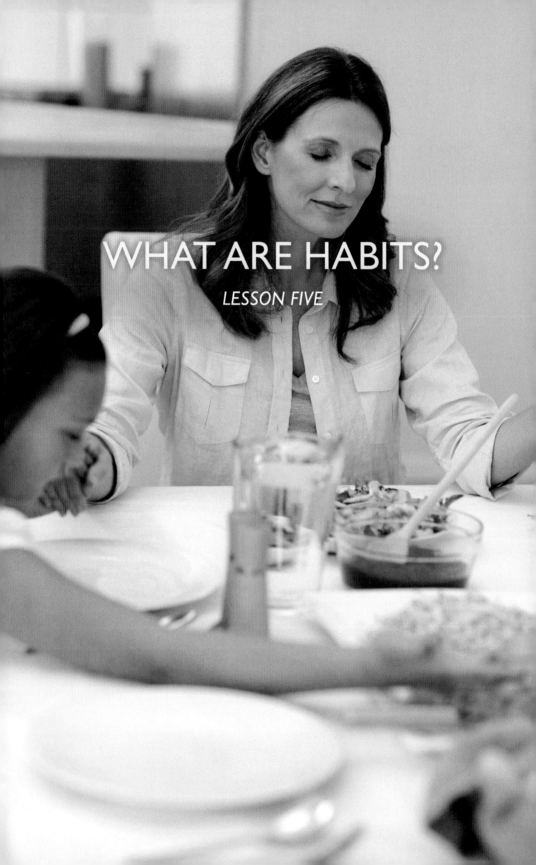

# WHAT ARE HABITS?

## LESSON FIVE

# WARM UP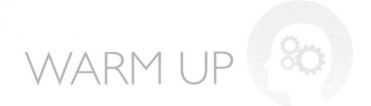

**Feedback: In what ways did God open the door since our last lesson for you to share some part of the lesson with someone else?**

.......................................................................................
.......................................................................................
.......................................................................................
.......................................................................................

Choose one or both questions to discuss (if in group setting)
or write out your answers on a separate sheet (for individual use):

1.  **What practical joke or prank are you most proud of doing?**[42]

.......................................................................................
.......................................................................................
.......................................................................................
.......................................................................................

2.  **What is one of your most satisfying accomplishments?**[43]

.......................................................................................
.......................................................................................
.......................................................................................
.......................................................................................

**Note to Reader:** *For the remaining lessons, which includes lessons 5-8 in part one, and the next series of 8 in part two, you will enter into a journey of discovery, learning how to incorporate into your life whatever new habits you choose to pursue. Each lesson will be another stepping stone to success, providing practical tools and insights for you to use.*

# DISCOVERY

We are all creatures of habit. The American Heritage Dictionary defines a habit, in part, as, "A constant, often unconscious inclination to perform an act, acquired through its frequent repetition."[44]

A pastor friend of mine accidently spilled some breakfast food on the white shirt he was wearing in preparation for his morning visits. Blueberry jam formed a dime-sized smudge under the left pocket. He finished eating then went into the bedroom to change shirts. He said that within five minutes, to his surprise, he was standing there fully outfitted in his blue, two-piece pajamas! In my humble opinion, that fits the definition of habit pretty well – "often unconscious inclination to perform an act." The neurons for undressing and the ones for going to bed were hard wired together in his head. While his thoughts were momentarily distracted by theological musings, habit simply took over even though it was at the wrong end of the day.

Habits, both good and bad, are at the center of who we are. The Scriptures have much to say about Bible characters who had various kinds of habits. For example:

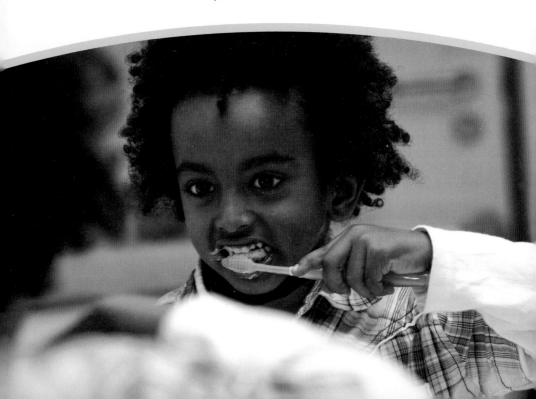

Jesus habitually prayed:

> "So He Himself often withdrew into the wilderness and prayed" (Luke 5:16, NKJV).

He went to the synagogue each week and taught:

> "And he came to Nazareth, where he had been brought up: and, as his custom was, he went into the synagogue on the Sabbath day, and stood up for to read" (Luke 4:16, NKJV).

Jesus always did what pleased his heavenly Father:

> "The one who sent me is with me; he has not left me alone, for I always do what pleases him" (John 8:29, NIV).

The disciples regularly praised God:

> "…and were continually in the temple praising and blessing God" (Luke 24:53, NKJV).

They also met together frequently in homes and ate together:

> "Every day they continued to meet together in the temple courts. They broke bread in their homes and ate together with glad and sincere hearts" (Acts 2:46, NIV).

Cornelius, a captain in the Italian Guard, often helped others and prayed:

> "He had led everyone in his house to live worshipfully before God, was always helping people in need, and had the habit of prayer" (Acts 10:2, MSG).

Tabitha made it a habit to help the poor:

> "In Joppa there was a disciple named Tabitha (in Greek her name is Dorcas); she was always doing good and helping the poor" (Acts 9:36, NIV).

The apostle Paul made it a habit to include thanksgiving in his prayers:

> ## "I always thank my God for you because of his grace given you in Christ Jesus."
>
> **1 CORINTHIANS 1:4, NIV**

Some bad habits are also acknowledged. For example:

Paul writes about some lazy gossips:

> *"Besides, they get into the habit of being idle and going about from house to house. And not only do they become idlers, but also busybodies who talk nonsense, saying things they ought not to"* (1 Timothy 5:13, NIV).

There are habits of *behavior*, and there are also habits of *thought*. There is the outward aspect of habits, but there is also the inner landscape of our minds with all of the complex mixture of thoughts and feelings. The two are very much related, because normally thoughts precede actions. *Both must be addressed if abundant living is to take root.*

In order to experience life to its fullest, there are two potential scenarios, (1) getting rid of bad habits, and (2) developing new ones.

*Actually, the very best way to do away with old habits is to replace them with better ones.* Jesus told a fascinating story in this regard. It might be likened to a scoundrel illegally inhabiting someone's vacant home that is up for sale. The police kick him out, but no guard is posted. Shortly the man is back with seven rascally friends and the situation is worse than ever, with raucous parties every night (Luke 11:24-26).

Focusing only on dumping old, scoundrelly habits can make us discouraged and we slip back into even worse behavior. Creating new habits to supplant them is much more motivating. The success principle here is displacement, the old adage of overcoming bad with good.

Bible scholar William Barclay makes the point well,

> *"The loveliest garden I ever saw was so full of flowers that there was scarcely room for a weed to grow. In no garden is it enough to uproot weeds; flowers must be sown and planted until the space is filled."*[45]

We may also, of course, create new habits that don't have any connection to any other previous habit at all.

The only way to obtain the increased happiness, effectiveness, and health you want for your life is through *habit and lifestyle change*. I certainly understand that the word "change" can send some people into nervous convulsions. "Oh no," they say, "anything but that!"

Suppose a mother butterfly is having one of those critical conversations with her young offspring Diane that all butterfly parents have to have at some point. Mom butterfly anticipates it with the same trepidation that most human parents experience before their inevitable, awkward talk with junior about the "birds and the bees."

This insect mother has glorious orange and black wings, sleek antennae, high cheek bones, and flowing brunette hair. Her daughter is still in the rather unimpressive, clunky, pre-teen caterpillar stage.

Mother informs her, "Someday soon you'll need to make a little chrysalis, a kind of windowless playhouse, get inside for several months, and when you come out you'll look a lot like me."[46]

The daughter pauses, looks down, then shakes her head and replies, "I'm going to do what?! Don't you like me the way I am?"

Mom tries to explain but is cut off.

"Look," Diane continues, "this 'chrysa' thing sounds really creepy. *Months* with no light? No food? No nectar? No friends? No phone or video games? Yuck!"

Like young Diane, we are, generally speaking, creatures of the status quo. Inertia, convenience, and our comfort level keep us clinging to the present. But we *can* enrich our lives. We *can* follow that inner voice that is calling us up higher. We *can* have our share of the abundant life that God longs for us to possess.

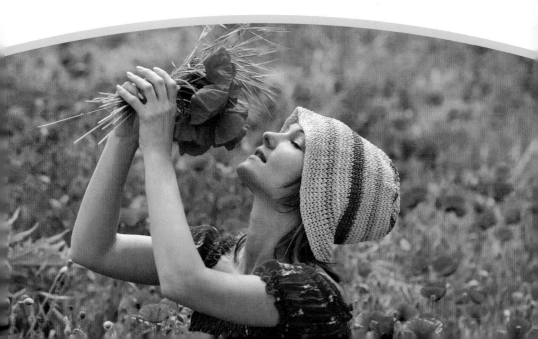

The two largest foundation stones for developing new habits and lifestyles are *Choice* and *Outlook*. Those two letters in the CREATION Health acronym form the underpinning for all other life change topics. They will be woven into the rest of the lessons in this series. Without slavishly repeating the two words, lessons 6–16 will nonetheless address those vital subjects from various angles and in various ways, integrating them throughout.

Choice *and* Outlook *are like the two blades of a kayak paddle. You need to utilize them both in order to get to your habit change destination.*

*Otherwise you just move in circles.*

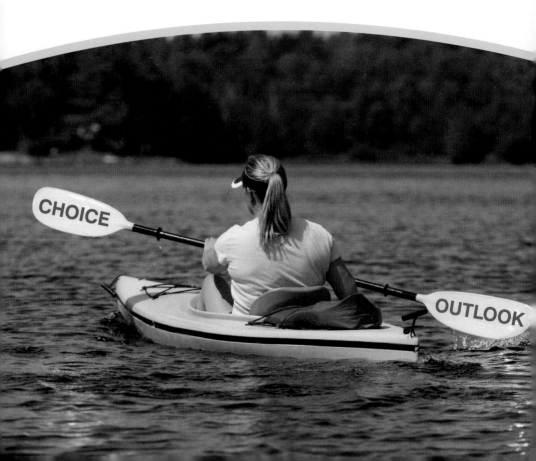

# CHOICE

Author and nationally known speaker, Hal Urban, observes,

> *"Millions of people are complaining about their lot, disgusted with life…and the way things are going, not realizing that there is a power which they possess which will permit them to take a new lease on life. Once you recognize this power and begin to use it, you can change your entire life and make it the way you would like to have it…filled with joy."* [47]

The power Urban refers to is the *power of choice*. It is a God-given gift that brings great possibilities and great responsibilities. When Adam and Eve were created, they were given the opportunity to choose good or evil. To be able to truly love, they needed to be free to decide on their own whether or not to serve God. Otherwise they would have been robots, parroting the responses their Creator programmed in. Free will, with all its attendant risks, was an absolute necessity. We have inherited that freedom and it is up to each of us to select the course of our lives, the journey we will pursue.

We are the CEO of our own life and happiness. We cannot abdicate that responsibility. It is built in. Comes with the territory. Even when we don't proactively choose, we are making a choice to be governed by outside forces and circumstances.

Today we are largely the sum of all our past decisions. Thankfully, the marvelous gift of choice means that the decisions of the past don't need to dictate our future. We can re-shape our lifestyle. We can create new habits. We can choose abundant living rather than merely surviving and existing. As William Jennings Bryan has well said, "Destiny is not a matter of chance. It is a matter of choice." [48]

> *"Destiny is not a matter of chance.*
> *It is a matter of choice."*
>
> **WILLIAM JENNINGS BRYAN**

# OUTLOOK

The dictionary definition of outlook is, "A point of view; attitude."[49] As the dictionary indicates, outlook is generally considered to be synonymous with attitude. It is our habitual way of viewing ourselves and the world around us. It is our inner interpretation of our surroundings.

The difference between a pessimistic attitude and an optimistic one is illustrated well by the epic story of David and Goliath. The Israelite soldiers looked at Goliath's enormous size and concluded they'd never be able to kill him. David looked at the very same giant and concluded, "He's so large there's no way I can miss."[50]

Just like any other choices we make in life, we can choose our outlook or attitude. When it comes to lifestyle change we can either be like the soldiers and conclude, "That challenge is way too much for me to handle." Or we can be like David and say, "Man, that's too big an opportunity to neglect."

One of the greatest barriers between you and the abundant life you yearn for is to get locked into old ways of thinking. Author and lecturer John Maxwell relates the following story,

> "I'm told that in northern Canada there are just two seasons: winter and July. When the back roads begin to thaw, they become muddy. Vehicles going into the backwoods country leave deep ruts that become frozen when cold weather returns. For those entering remote areas during the winter months, there are signs that read, 'Driver, please choose carefully which rut you drive in, because you'll be in it for the next twenty miles.' Some people seem to feel stuck in their current attitudes like a car in a twenty mile rut. However, attitude is not permanent. If you're not happy with yours, know that you can change."[51]

## "The Lord is with me; I will not be afraid."

**PSALM 118:6, NIV**

CREATION HEALTH | LIFE GUIDE #1

We don't have to remain in a rut and declare, "Well, that's just the way I am." When it comes to developing new habits, openness to change and optimism regarding our success are vital. An attitude of hopefulness is also one of the keys that keeps us moving forward.

Our outlook often determines our choices and our choices, in turn, reflexively impact our outlook. They are related and work together to take us into the future we desire. It is that future that Dawna Markova addresses in her thought-provoking question, "Am I living the life that wants to live in me?"[52]

It is encouraging to know that you do not need to pursue your habit change journey alone. God promises to be your partner and provide tremendous spiritual resources. Choosing to avail ourselves of his assistance will enable our outlook to be full of hope and optimism. We can say with the Psalmist, "The Lord is with me; I will not be afraid" (Psalm 118:6, NIV).

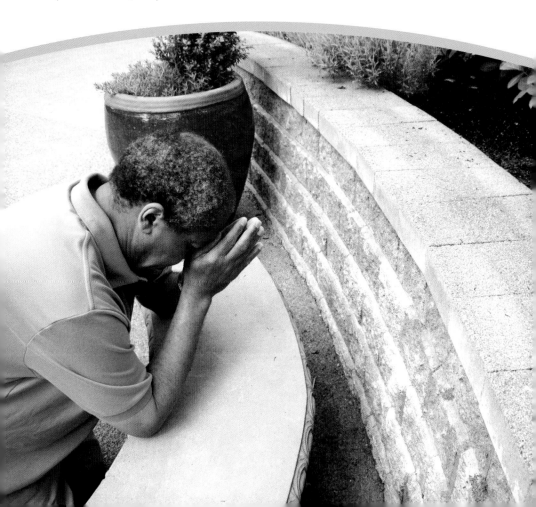

# DISCUSSION

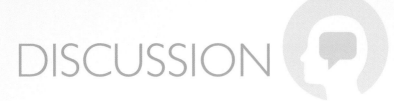

Can you think of other Bible characters who had good or bad habits?

......................................................................................

......................................................................................

What do you think is included in the phrase "habits of thinking"?

......................................................................................

......................................................................................

How do you normally relate to personal change?

......................................................................................

......................................................................................

How have habits formed in your own life?

......................................................................................

......................................................................................

What ruts of attitude are you most likely to slip into?

......................................................................................

......................................................................................

How can we tell when we are in a rut in our thinking?

......................................................................................

......................................................................................

If you were David's best friend, what advice would you have given him when you heard that he wanted to confront Goliath?

......................................................................................

......................................................................................

If you are CEO of your own life, how would you describe your management style? What grade would you give yourself over the last six months?

......................................................................................

......................................................................................

How do you perceive Outlook and Choice working together to form habits?

......................................................................................

......................................................................................

# SHARING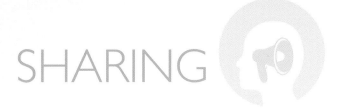

## OPPORTUNITY #5:

- Pray as a group for God to open the way for you to share something from these lessons to help someone else.

- Keep your radar up each day for opportunities.

### ABUNDANT LIVING THOUGHT

Our outlook often determines our choices and our choices, in turn, reflexively impact our outlook. They are related and work together to take us into the future we desire. It is that future that Dawna Markova addresses in her thought-provoking question, "Am I living the life that wants to live in me?"

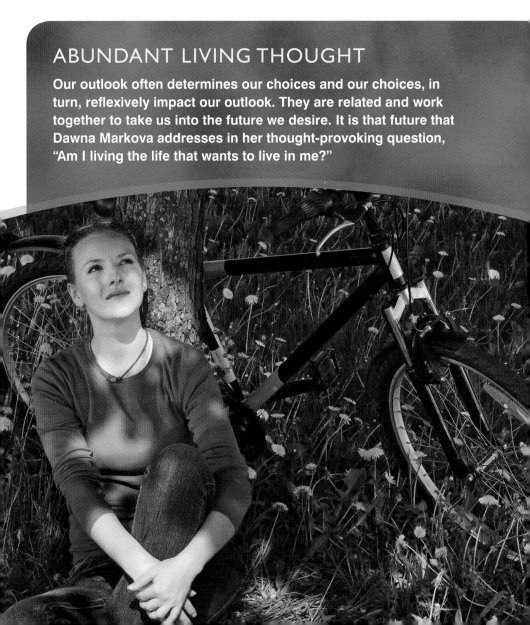

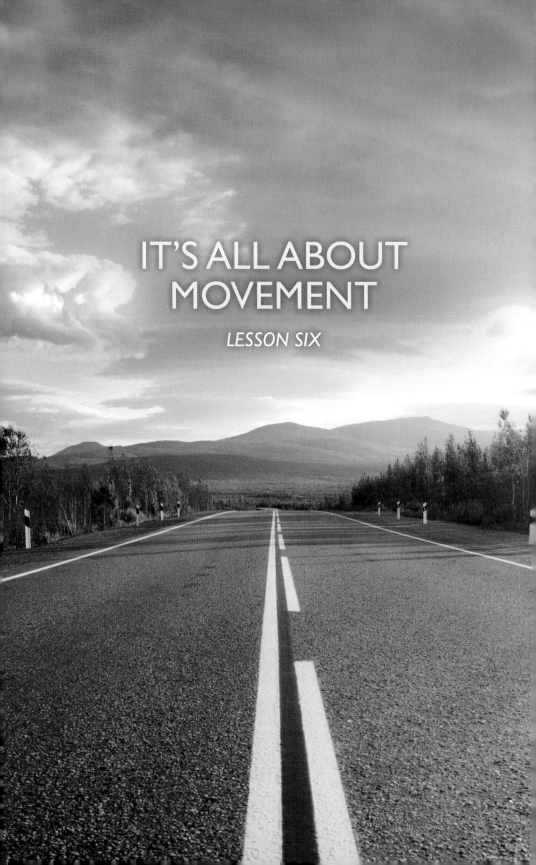

# IT'S ALL ABOUT MOVEMENT

*LESSON SIX*

# WARM UP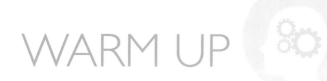

**Feedback: In what ways did God open the door since our last lesson for you to share some part of the lesson with someone else?**

..........................................................................
..........................................................................
..........................................................................
..........................................................................

Choose one or both questions to discuss (if in group setting) or write out your answers on a separate sheet (for individual use):

1. **What caused you to feel overwhelmed recently?[53] Describe the event.**

..........................................................................
..........................................................................
..........................................................................
..........................................................................

2. **What event or experience from the past made you feel awe and/or amazement?[54]**

..........................................................................
..........................................................................
..........................................................................
..........................................................................

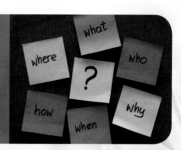

*"In short, you decide your destiny by the daily choices you make."*

**DR. DICK TIBBITS**

# DISCOVERY

The process of habit creation is a lot like a road trip vacation our family took. It was a journey from Maine headed west through the northern tier of states on Route 90, then dropping down into Colorado and Utah, taking a hard left turn after Arizona on Route 40, heading back along the southern route and finally up into Virginia and a bunch of other states on the Eastern seaboard.

From the beginning we intended on completing the 3,000 mile circuit, but we had much to celebrate all along the way because our larger purpose was for each of us to grow. That could happen in all kinds of ways such as awareness of the diversity that is America, appreciation for the wonders of nature, and making memories together. We were growing *every day* through experiences such as the hurricane force winds that nearly destroyed our tent, the hike into the snow capped Rockies, the mule ride down the Grand Canyon, the "Trail of Tears" outdoor dramatization of the plight of the Cherokee Indians, to name a few. If we had focused the whole time only on getting home we would have missed so much and the travel itself would have been viewed as an obstacle and drudgery rather than a fantastic opportunity.

Likewise, success in habit creation should not simply be measured by the point at which you arrive at a particular end destination such as regularly exercising five times a week or getting seven or eight hours of sleep. Habit formation is a journey. By comparing it to a vacation I don't mean to imply that it is a piece of cake. Not usually. *But, like a vacation, it is a process within which you can succeed all along the way if you know what to look for.* Focusing on the journey itself doesn't lessen interest in achieving a particular change; it actually makes it much more likely that you'll get there.

The concept of viewing lifestyle change as a journey is the central theme of a groundbreaking book entitled *Changing for Good.*[55] The authors identify six separate and distinct stages in the process of habit formation. People move through these stages in their pursuit of a higher level of wholeness and satisfaction. There are no short-cuts. No one stage is more important than any other. Each stage is important and contributes to advancing the journey.

What follows is a brief overview of each of these six elements, called Prochaska's six stages.

## 1. Precontemplation

This is the stage when a person doesn't want to change. They see no problem with the status quo. If change involves giving up some long cherished habit, they will often retreat into denial or rationalization.

This is not the time to nag, harass, or hassle someone to change. This is not the time to say, "You're so hard headed and stubborn!" It only gets them to dig their heels in deeper.

So what can help get them to modify their behavior? Life events, transitions, and milestones such as moving, marriage, divorce, childbirth, graduations, and illness are often triggers and can provide the needed push. Pressure from society can also help, such as the media calling attention to the dangers of obesity or smoking. Maintaining a close, non-judgmental attitude allows helpers to remain approachable when someone in the precontemplation stage does start thinking about the possibility of change.[56]

If you are currently in this stage, one of the best things you can do is to increase your awareness of the problem and potential risks and solutions.

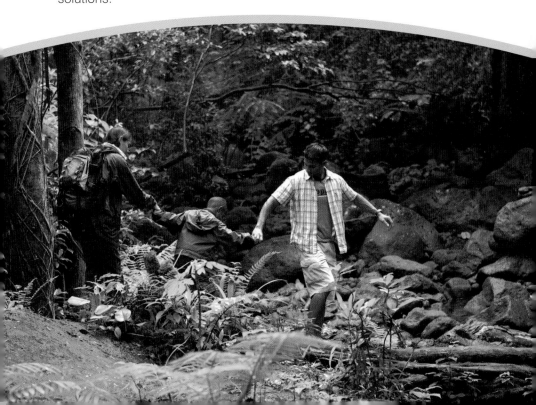

## 2.  Contemplation

In this stage, individuals start to think seriously about change. It is not definite, but it's at least on the radar. They are ambivalent, but that's OK because all they really need is fifty-one percent, a majority vote from their own mind, to get started.

One of the key questions to be asked at this stage is, "What is the payoff of the old habit?" It may be psychological or physical, and might include such things as pleasure and control. Whatever the payoff is, it has to be replaced by the new habit or else we will be sucked back into old patterns. Listing the advantages of a new habit is also essential in order to make it attractive enough to overcome the current inertia.[57]

## 3.  Preparation

Most people in this stage are convinced of the need to change, have given it serious reflection, maybe even researched the topic, and now anticipate adopting the new habit within the next month or so. They take the time to develop a game plan that includes time frames and strategies for implementation. A strong commitment is essential here. At this point, the anticipated change gets moved high up the priority list.[58]

Notice that these first three stages are all *internal*. They deal with what's happening inside the brain, because all habit change begins with re-orienting our thinking. Trying to change one's actions without first changing their thought processes and perspective is doomed to failure. As the Scriptures indicate, "As he thinks in his heart, so is he" (Proverbs 23:7, NKJV).

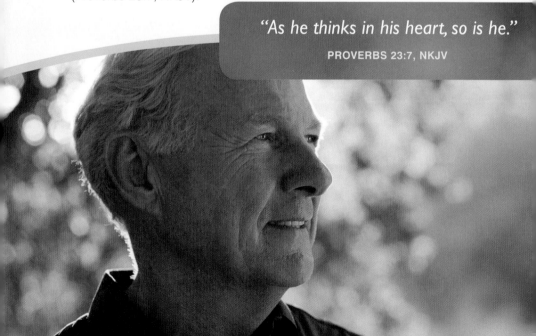

"As he thinks in his heart, so is he."

PROVERBS 23:7, NKJV

## 4. Action

As the label indicates, individuals in this stage act on their commitments and plans. They make changes in both thinking and outward behavior. This is the stage that requires the most time and energy. During this part of the journey, people learn to deal with urges and relapses through diversion, exercise, relaxation, self-talk, learning to say "No," restructuring their environment, rewarding themselves, recalling their vision and purpose, reviewing advantages and disadvantages, and, most of all, plugging into divine power.[59]

## 5. Maintenance

At this stage people need to work to consolidate their gains and deepen the lifestyle change they have adopted.

## 6. Termination

Here a person has lived with their new habit for so long that it has become second nature and any former urges or lapses are no longer an issue.

Failure to achieve habit change is often the result of going directly to the *action* stage without spending time in the foundational stages that lead up to it.

Focusing only on action is like a peculiar, imaginary school that focuses only on final exams. Students pay $25,000 to take a full load of classes toward their bachelor's degree. The bulletin lists all of the many courses and professors. The school calendar, however, indicates that college is only open the first week of each semester for finals. No lectures. No homework. No research papers. No interaction with professors. No learning. No preparation. No foundation. Just take the exam. Sink or swim.

It is not unlike that to skip over the early, internal stages of change. The likelihood of success is very limited.

The great news in the stages of habit creation is that we can experience success at many points during our lifestyle change journey. Someone who moves from *precontemplation* to *contemplation* has made tremendous progress even though no outward change can yet be seen. Research indicates that people often get stuck for years in *contemplation*. So when they then move to the next stage, *preparation* and planning, they have much to rejoice about. If someone asked them, "So how is your new lifestyle coming?" they could legitimately answer, "Terrific," even though they have made no alterations as yet in their behavior. Not only can they find cause for encouragement as they move through Prochaska's six stages, they can also find things to celebrate within each stage. Such feelings of success are critical because they build momentum, fuel motivation, and inspire hope.

What would it be like to apply these six stages of change to Bible characters? One that comes to mind is a man named Zacchaeus.

*"Then Jesus entered and walked through Jericho. There was a man there, his name Zacchaeus, the head tax man and quite rich. He wanted desperately to see Jesus, but the crowd was in his way – he was a short man and couldn't see over the crowd. So he ran on ahead and climbed up in a sycamore tree so he could see Jesus when he came by" (Luke 19:1-4, MSG).*

Zacchaeus was the wealthy director of the Jericho tax bureau. Employed by Rome, he, along with his fellow tax men, was notorious for extortion of the masses. Hated is an understatement. Living high, he had no interest in change and laughed off any such suggestion [*precontemplation*].

Before Jesus' visit, reports had undoubtedly filtered back to Zacchaeus of the preaching of John the Baptist, who admonished such tax collectors specifically, "Exact no more than that which is appointed you" (Luke 3:13, KJV). For the first time, conviction gripped his heart [*contemplation*].

Zacchaeus then heard that, remarkably, Christ had chosen a Roman tax collector as one of his twelve disciples (Matthew 10:3). Jesus also befriended and ate with members of the despised profession (Matthew 9:10). In those days it was unheard of for a rabbi to do such a thing. Such grace and acceptance inspired the little man to reach higher and create a very different lifestyle. He chose to change [*preparation*].

When Jesus and his followers unexpectedly walked through downtown Jericho, Zacchaeus became so convicted that he forgot his normally high brow bearing and scurried up a tree for a better view. Christ halted under its branches, looked up, called the infamous extortioner by name, and invited himself to the man's home for dinner.

The invitation shocked Zacchaeus and he instantly made good on his commitment to a new life, announcing an astonishing, self-imposed remedy – "Here and now I give *half* of my possessions to the poor, and if I have cheated anybody out of anything, I will pay back *four times* the amount" (Luke 19:8, NIV) [*action*].

As a result, Jesus gladly announced that salvation had now come to Zacchaeus and his whole family, which indicates that this was not a temporary commitment, but a new, ongoing lifestyle (Luke 19:9) [*maintenance and termination*].

With divine intervention, Zacchaues' habit creation journey took him from being a miserly Scrooge to becoming a habitually gracious, happy philanthropist.

Our own journey will not be so dramatic, but the tax collector's major makeover can nonetheless be instructive and inspiring.

Zacchaeus moved through the stages of change in order, one after the next. Research indicates, however, that many people's journey through the various stages is not linear like that. They don't just move in a forward direction. Sometimes they cycle back, for instance from *Action* to *Contemplation*, catch their breath, regroup, and then advance again. Each person finds their own rhythm, pace, and direction. Moving through the six stages of habit development can be a great source of encouragement as we become more aware of our own progress.

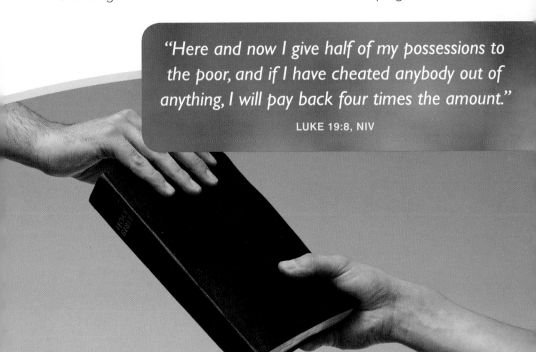

"*Here and now I give half of my possessions to the poor, and if I have cheated anybody out of anything, I will pay back four times the amount.*"

LUKE 19:8, NIV

M.J. Ryan provides another source of encouragement by identifying *three key phases of learning* during habit creation that mark tremendous progress as well. The phases are called (pardon the Latin), (1) Post Hoc, (2) Ad Hoc, and (3) Pre Hoc.[60]

1.  In ***Post Hoc*** **learning, we recognize** *after the fact* **that we wanted to do something differently. We say things like, "Oh no, I forgot to eat my veggies at lunch."**

2.  In ***Ad Hoc***, **we recognize** *while we're eating lunch* **that we didn't include veggies.**

3.  In ***Pre Hoc***, **we recognize** *prior to eating lunch* **that we need to include veggies.**

Moving from one phase of learning to the next is certainly cause for commendation. Even *Post Hoc* is progress over not sensing any need for veggies at all. These are largely internal changes that will most likely not be noticed by others.

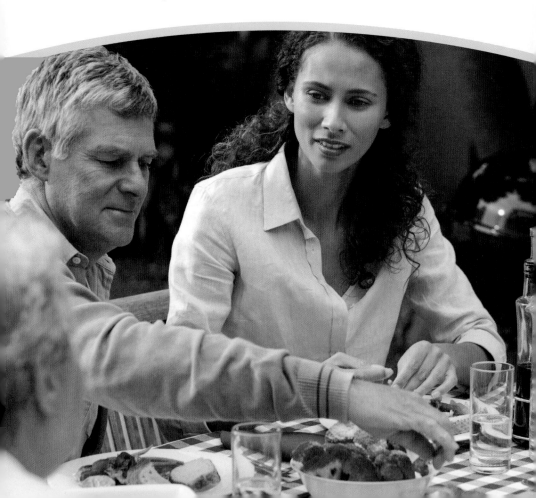

More encouragement can be found in, of all places, *our failures*. The word "failure" needs to be re-examined because there can be plenty of reason for celebration here as well.

1. **Failure is a positive if we learn from it.**

2. **Failure is a positive if it means we have stretched beyond our current capabilities. In fact, lack of failure is probably a sign that we are not stretching ourselves enough.**

3. **Failure is a positive if we get up, shake ourselves off, and have the courage to keep moving forward. We are always stronger as a result.**

M. J. Ryan writes, "If I could leave you with only one tip for changing anything in your life, it would be this, *recognizing you've blown it is progress!*"[61]

The emphasis in this chapter on some of the many ways we can label our efforts a success as we pursue new lifestyle habits is not Polyannish or naïve. There certainly can be periods of disappointment, discouragement, and exhaustion. This chapter is an attempt to re-orient our thinking and provide us with a new perspective on reality that sees formerly hidden sources of hope. It tries to help us look deeper for the "story behind the story" and give us legitimate reasons to pat ourselves on the back as we take each new, sometimes halting, often shaky, step forward.

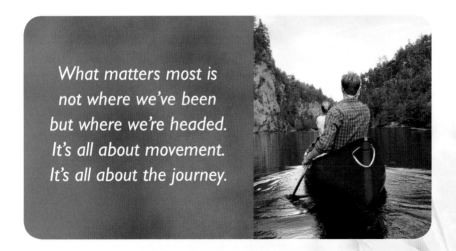

*What matters most is not where we've been but where we're headed. It's all about movement. It's all about the journey.*

# DISCUSSION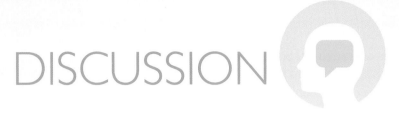

Have you ever been resistant to change in the precontemplation stage? Did anyone try to get you to change?

........................................................................................................

........................................................................................................

Are you in either the contemplation or preparation stage for some potential change in your life? What would that change be like for you?

........................................................................................................

........................................................................................................

Why do we tend to pay so much attention to the action stage to the near exclusion of any others?

........................................................................................................

........................................................................................................

How does knowing about the Prochaska's six stages alter your view of people who are struggling to change?

........................................................................................................

........................................................................................................

If you could listen in on Zacchaeus' thoughts as he pondered how much money to return to the victims and the poor, what would he be thinking?

........................................................................................................

........................................................................................................

What do you find most encouraging about the concept of *Post Hoc, Ad Hoc*, and *Pre Hoc*?

........................................................................................................

........................................................................................................

What adjustment do you need to make in your thinking to view failure as a positive?

........................................................................................................

........................................................................................................

What sources of hope does this chapter provide for you in the area of habit change?

........................................................................................................

........................................................................................................

........................................................................................................

# SHARING

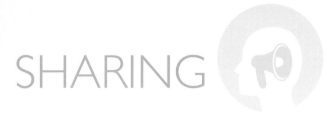

## OPPORTUNITY #6:

- Pray as a group for God to open the way for you to share something from these lessons to help someone else.

- Keep your radar up each day for opportunities.

**How this lesson can impact our Choices and Outlook**

CHOICE:

1. We can choose to be proactive about change rather than being reactive to events.

2. The choices we make at each stage of habit change either keep us moving forward or cause us to stagnate.

OUTLOOK:

1. We can view change as a journey and a movement through stages rather than a one-time event.

2. With the right attitude, we can find much to celebrate as we create new habits.

## ABUNDANT LIVING THOUGHT

M. J. Ryan writes, "If I could leave you with only one tip for changing anything in your life, it would be this, recognizing you've blown it is progress!"

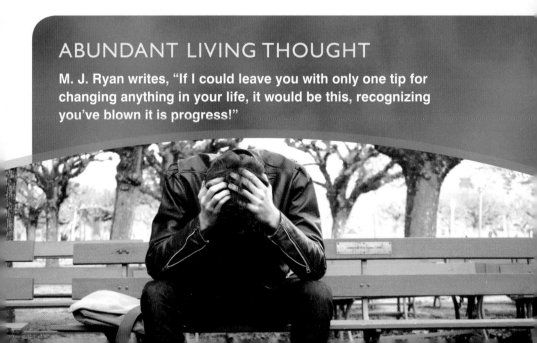

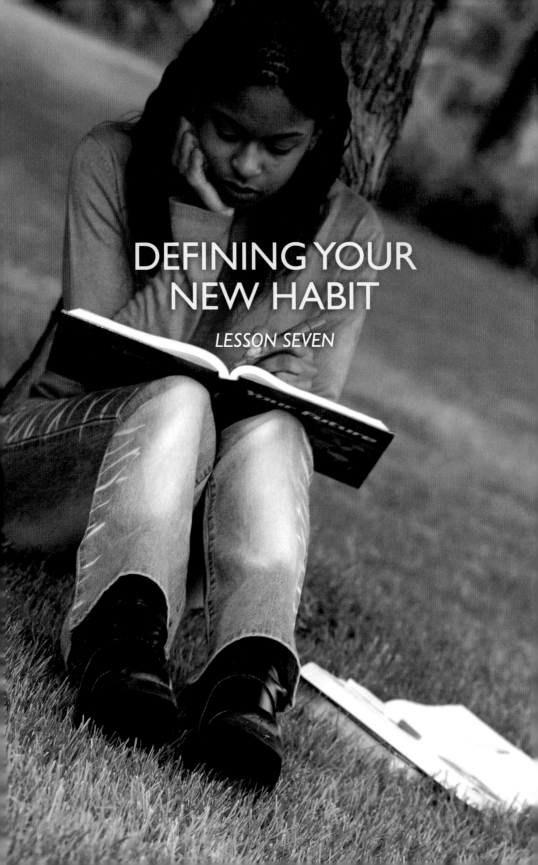

# DEFINING YOUR NEW HABIT

## LESSON SEVEN

# WARM UP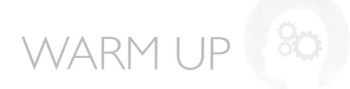

**Feedback: In what ways did God open the door since our last lesson for you to share some part of the lesson with someone else?**

..........................................................................................................
..........................................................................................................
..........................................................................................................
..........................................................................................................

Choose one or both questions to discuss (if in group setting)
or write out your answers on a separate sheet (for individual use):

1.  **Would anyone like to share what's been happening in their habit development journey?**

..........................................................................................................
..........................................................................................................
..........................................................................................................
..........................................................................................................

2.  **Would you characterize your past week as sunny, partly cloudy, mostly cloudy, or stormy? Why?**

..........................................................................................................
..........................................................................................................
..........................................................................................................
..........................................................................................................

> *"Choosing with thought and intention is your greatest power."*
> MONICA REED, MD

# DISCOVERY

It's time now to start defining the new habit(s) you want to create. It is probably best to limit yourself to developing one new habit at a time, but that is up to you. There is truth in the old adage: *"Be like a postage stamp - stick to one thing until you get there."*[62]

You want to move beyond the typical short-lived New Year's Resolution and focus on something you can permanently and successfully build into your life. *In order for that to happen, this lesson provides some essential guidelines for selecting and defining your new habit.* It may be something intended to counteract an old habit, or it may be something completely unrelated to an old habit at all.

Nonetheless, the more thoughtfully you choose, the better. We want to move from a choice that is whimsical to one that is very intentional; from one that is spur of the moment to one that is the product of careful reflection. Give yourself the gift of paying attention to your own happiness and fulfillment. Without question, you're worth it!

The closer you can align your choice of a new habit with the following guidelines, the greater the potential for success.

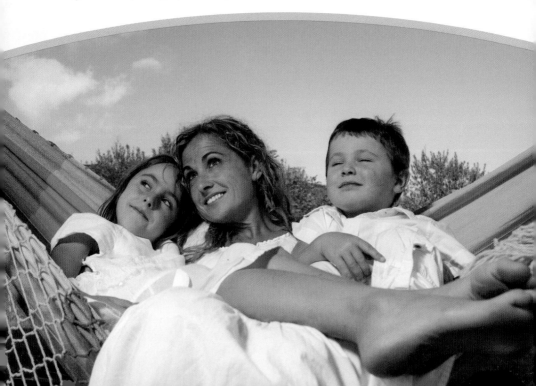

1. **First decide what area of life you want to focus on. There are various areas where new habits could emerge:**

## Your Own Personal Growth

It might be physical, mental, emotional, or spiritual growth that involves reading, taking classes, traveling, receiving counseling, undertaking certain pursuits, etc. You may even have a deep sense of calling to a new avocation.

I remember when I first felt the inner stirring to write. As a professional accountant, my days were consumed with numbers, making sure all of the debits equaled those pesky credits. I sensed a vague pull, a tug on my heart and mind, to put pen to paper and share my perspectives on God and spiritual living. After that initial stirring came insistent messages from the Naysayer Department of my brain – *"YOU, a WRITER! You've got to be kidding. That's absurd. How are you going to find time and, besides, who would care anything about what you have to say anyway?"* It was bad. I told God, "I'll give writing my best shot for two years. If doors open, I'll keep walking through them. If not, I'll chalk up the tug on my heart to heartburn." That's almost fifteen years ago and I'm still writing.

So if there is a dream sprouting within your heart, get feedback from people who care about you, make adjustments as needed, then water that little seed and help it grow to become an important part of your life.

## Your Growth in Relationship to Others

Everyone has both primary relationships with family and close friends, and secondary relationships with neighbors, co-workers, church members, etc. Any of these is a fertile area for new habits to develop.

Several years ago I had to make a significant adjustment in how I discussed issues with my wife, especially as they related to our marriage or the house. One day she raised the issue of me needing to clean up the garage. My knee-jerk reaction was to instantly debate.

She'd say, "Kim, it makes me feel very unsettled when the garage is so cluttered."

"Cluttered? It's not cluttered at all. Ask me for anything out there and I can find it with no problem whatsoever."

"But everything is soooo scattered."

"Everything? You're saying that *everything* is just tossed around out there, huh? My wrenches are in perfect order. The old tires are piled up nicely."

"But you never take time to clean up after yourself."

"Never? I've *never* cleaned up anything out there? *Nothing*? How about the time I took that old paint down to the Recycle Center? Then there's the old sneakers I tossed. You call that nothing?"

On and on. Needless to say, this behavior on my part was not at all helpful. Nothing "abundant living" about it. So I eventually decided to change. Not easy, but I don't debate much anymore. I learned to listen a whole lot better. I also learned that the issue that wives bring up initially is not always the *real* issue. By God's grace, I altered my habitual way of relating.

**Your involvement in community organizations and causes is another area for new habits to develop**

Many people feel there's a lack of real purpose in their lives. They are experiencing financial and professional success, but there is a deep longing to be caught up in something larger than themselves, some selfless service with no expectation of reward. They feel drawn to help others but aren't sure where to begin. Simply contacting local agencies or searching online for non-profit organizations and contacting them can spark the creation of habits of altruism that last a lifetime.

2. **Your new habit needs to be abundant living oriented (see Lessons 2-4).**

Focus primarily on what you are *adding* to your life, not what you are *subtracting*. Abundant living does not have much to do with money or even circumstances. It is mostly about adopting ways of thinking and behaving that bring more fullness, holistic health, and effectiveness into our lives. It is about living proactively and not reactively. It is about taking back control and setting an intentional course toward greater well-being and satisfaction.

> *Focus on what you are adding to your life, not what you are subtracting.*

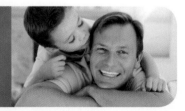

## 3. The new habit needs to be something you value enough to stay with it, to make it happen.

The best way to discover what new habit you have the best chance of sticking with long term is to make sure it is *firmly rooted in your values.* Your values can be defined as, *"What we believe to be of greatest importance and of highest priority in our lives."*[63] Values get at what makes each of us distinctive in this world.

Here are some questions that can help you discover what is most valuable in your life:

> *What is most important to me in each of my roles and relationships?*
>
> *What do I like to do most in my spare time?*
>
> *What do I enjoy sharing with others?*
>
> *What do I want my children to be like? Your example will be the most powerful influence on their behavior.*
>
> *When I look back at the end of my life, what will I be glad that I did?*
>
> *What am I doing when I feel most fulfilled and/or joyful?*
>
> *What am I willing to pour my energies into?*
>
> *What would cause me the greatest sense of loss if it was not in my life?*[64]

One of the best indicators of our true values is the way we spend our time. It is not what we say or intend but what we actually do that reveals our deepest loyalties and commitments. When I say, "I don't have time," I am, in essence, saying that I value something else more.

Jesus' life was clearly values-driven. He summarized those values while visiting the synagogue where he grew up in his hometown of Nazareth. Opening the scroll of the Old Testament book Isaiah, Christ read from Isaiah 61 and applied its words to himself:

> *"The Spirit of the LORD is upon Me,*
> *Because He has anointed Me*
> *To preach the gospel to the poor;*
> *He has sent Me to heal the brokenhearted,*
> *To proclaim liberty to the captives*
> *And recovery of sight to the blind,*
> *To set at liberty those who are oppressed;*
> *To proclaim the acceptable year of the LORD" (Luke 4:18-19, NKJV).*

These values led Christ to make a major career change, leave home, live off donations, sleep under the stars, visit hundreds of villages, and eventually become a martyr. I'm sure he re-read these verses often and taught them fervently to his disciples. Here was the North Star of Jesus' life and ministry.

The apostle Paul also led a value-centered life. The supreme value for the great missionary was to spread the Gospel. In 1 Corinthians, he states,

> *"For I decided to know nothing among you except Jesus Christ and him crucified" (1 Corinthians 2:2, RSV).*

This value compelled him to put his life at risk time and time again for the sake of Jesus. He spent years in dank, filthy prisons, was shipwrecked, flogged, beaten, assaulted, and stoned.

It is all too human for our values and behavior to get out of sync and not match up in one way or another. When that happens we can feel unsettled, uneasy, anxious, unfulfilled. *It can often be the case that we are not able to keep a new habit resolution because we value something more that interferes with it.* If we don't recognize when that is happening, we can be disappointed in our own lack of success.[65]

4.  **Your new habit needs to be something you can picture in your mind, a mental image.**
One of the most successful ways to accomplish lifestyle change is create a clear mental picture of the change you desire *and then live into it*. The sharper the vision, the better able you are to make it a reality.[66]

One suggestion is to write yourself a letter from the you who will be living your new habit one year from now. Imagine yourself after you have accomplished your plan, your resolution. There you are! It's the future you who has slimmed down, eaten healthier, learned to relax, fixed the problem in a relationship, realized how to trust God more fully, adopted a more optimistic attitude, become more active, built a network of friends, taken on that hobby, or joined that non-profit cause.

In your mind, try to picture your future self as clearly and realistically as possible. What are you wearing? What is your expression? Where are you? What are you feeling? What are you saying? What are you doing? *What can that future self say to you now about how to get there?*[67]

It is that mental image that gives you clarity, focus, motivation, definition, and a target to shoot for.

That image also needs to become part of your self-identity *now*. For me to become a runner, I have to picture myself doing that first and incorporate it into my identity *before* I earn that label by actually running. It can feel hypocritical, but it is nonetheless essential. When I don't run, I remind myself, "Hey, I'm a runner; I need to get out there." Whatever new habit you want to incorporate into your life, *be* it in your mind before you *are* actually in it. The actions you choose to take flow out from that new self-understanding.

### 5. Your new habit needs to be compelling and hook into your feelings.

Researchers have discovered that, contrary to most people's approach to personal change, we do not usually change because of information alone. People who attain success are far more likely to take information and analyze it, *but then go further by linking it up with something that evokes positive emotions.*[68]

It is vital that the new person we want to become grabs our feelings because *good feelings get us moving and keep us moving.* It doesn't mean that we are giddy, but that our emotions are engaged enough to get our attention and fuel our journey forward.* It's the difference between "Drive 400 miles a day" and "Travel to Disney World." The latter gets us driving and powers up our motivation to go the distance.

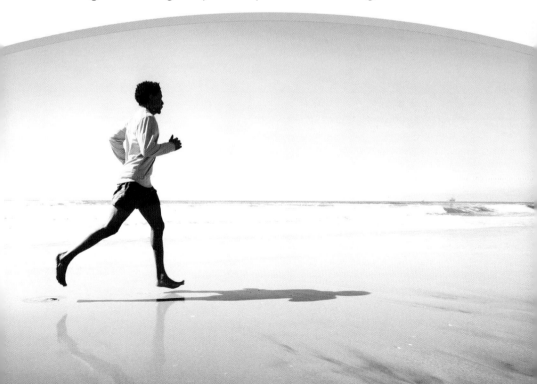

The examples below pull together several key elements from this lesson and show how our values and mental image can connect to our feelings. The column on the left contains worthwhile habits that are, nonetheless, boring and unmotivating and unlikely to be sustained. The column on the right creates a mental image that hooks into our feelings and fuels the daily change we desire in a sustainable way.

| Boring/Unmotivating | Energizing/Motivating |
| --- | --- |
| Write three pages every day | Holding my first published book in my hands. |
| Run four days per week | Crossing the finish line at two 10K runs each year. |
| Eat veggies five times a week | My family asking for "More veggies please." |
| Stop interrupting my wife | My wife smiles as I let her know how much I care by listening carefully. |
| Get to bed by 10 p.m. | I wake up with energy and optimism each day. |
| Do your night school homework | Masters degree in hand, I begin my new career. |
| Stop eating cookies every night | See myself fitting into a great new outfit. |
| Read my Bible everyday | Feel a new sense of spiritual peace and joy flowing into my life. |
| Get home from work earlier | Rolling around on the floor with my kids as we laugh together. |
| Don't watch so much TV | Participating in a ministry that helps displaced families. |
| Stop worrying so much | Encouraging someone else at a local support group for overcoming fear and anxiety. |
| Stop berating yourself | I will treat myself the way I imagine Jesus treating me. |

When you finally define your new habit, it is very important to *write it down.* Sounds like a hassle, but that simple act can greatly increase your potential for success. Get it down, keep it handy, and refer to it often.

*The exception is when change is doctor prescribed regarding a critical health issue. In that case we need to follow orders regardless of how we feel about it.*

## Group exercise
Brainstorm possibilities for filling in the right column:

| Boring/Unmotivating | Energizing/Motivating |
|---|---|
| Clean the house every week | |
| Weed the garden | |
| Eat less salt | |
| **Fill in your suggestions:** | |

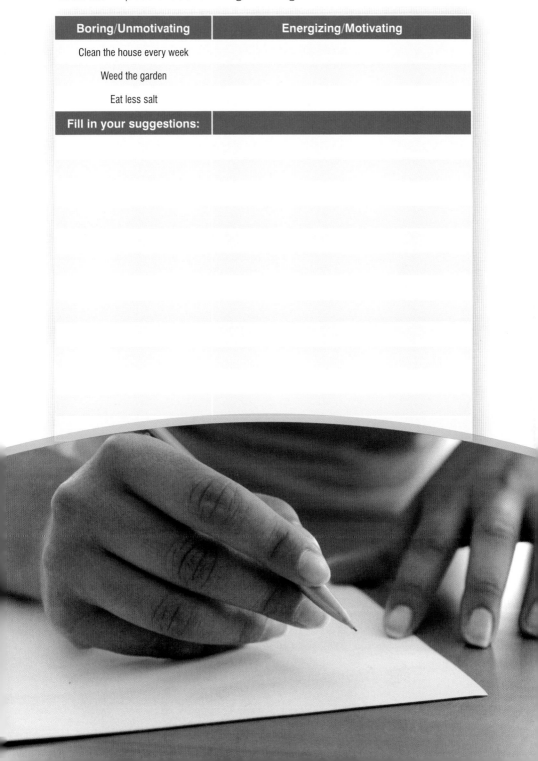

# DISCUSSION

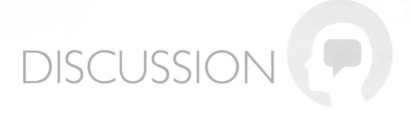

In what area of your life would you consider creating a new habit? What might that habit look like?

.............................................................................................................
.............................................................................................................

In your opinion, what is one of the most important habits for maintaining healthy relationships? Where are you in relation to that habit?

.............................................................................................................
.............................................................................................................

What do you feel is your primary purpose in life?

.............................................................................................................
.............................................................................................................

Which abundant living habit caught your attention the most from Lessons 2-4?

.............................................................................................................
.............................................................................................................

How would you summarize Jesus' values, as expressed in Luke 4, in a four-word sentence?

.............................................................................................................
.............................................................................................................

What are your top three values in life? Why did you choose them?

.............................................................................................................
.............................................................................................................

What does the way you spend your time tell you about your value system?

.............................................................................................................
.............................................................................................................

Describe a mental image you have of a better you.

.............................................................................................................
.............................................................................................................

From the list of unmotivating and motivating habit definitions at the end of the lesson, which one captures your interest the most? Why?

.............................................................................................................
.............................................................................................................

.............................................................................................................

# SHARING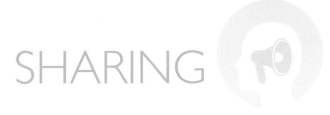

## OPPORTUNITY #7:

- Pray as a group for God to open the way for you to share something from these lessons to help someone else.

- Keep your radar up each day for opportunities.

**How this lesson can impact our Choices and Outlook**

CHOICE:

1. Choosing what habit to create should be based on certain guidelines.

2. We choose our values which become the foundation for change.

OUTLOOK:

1. For change to be successful, we need to be able to envision a positive outcome from our efforts.

2. We have to allow change to impact our feelings and not simply our logical mind.

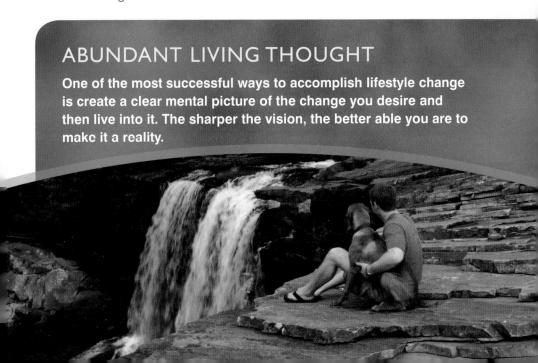

## ABUNDANT LIVING THOUGHT

**One of the most successful ways to accomplish lifestyle change is create a clear mental picture of the change you desire and then live into it. The sharper the vision, the better able you are to make it a reality.**

# SMALL STEPS
# ARE A BIG DEAL

## *LESSON EIGHT*

# WARM UP

**Feedback: In what ways did God open the door since our last lesson for you to share some part of the lesson with someone else?**

.........................................................................................
.........................................................................................
.........................................................................................
.........................................................................................

Choose one or both questions to discuss (if in group setting)
or write out your answers on a separate sheet (for individual use):

1. **What hobbies do you enjoy?**[69]

.........................................................................................
.........................................................................................
.........................................................................................
.........................................................................................

2. **In what ways has your life been changing while studying these lessons?**

.........................................................................................
.........................................................................................
.........................................................................................
.........................................................................................

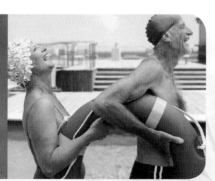

*"Allow the world
to live as it chooses,
and allow yourself
to live as you choose."*

**RICHARD BACH**

# DISCOVERY

Now that you have arrived at a definition of your new habit from lesson 7, it is time to start thinking about how to get there, how to turn a vision into reality. *You do that by setting and achieving goals.* Goals are the stepping stones to your abundant living future.

Imagine you have chosen to enter a five mile race. It is scheduled for 8:00 a.m. as one of the events in the annual 4th of July celebration. Your family and several close friends are standing near the start line to offer support. You have purchased new shorts and sneakers for the occasion and been given the number 435 emblazoned on a handkerchief sized piece of orange cloth draped across your chest. You amble nervously up to the start line surrounded by several hundred eager runners. Scanning the other entrants, you try hard to stay within yourself, focusing only on your own goals and performance. At 7:57 a.m. it is already warm. You pull the visor on your baseball cap down further on your sweat tinged forehead.

The large digital display nearby clicks down the time. 7:58. 7:59. You tense, peer down the road ahead, and lean forward slightly. Cheers and clapping begin to escalate. The excitement is palpable. Suddenly the gun fires and everyone surges forward. *You take one, deliberate step, stop, and then throw up your hands in joyous celebration.* Your family rushes out to hug you. Together you make your way back to the car and the wonderful backyard barbecue that awaits.

Odd? For sure, but I exaggerated so the illustration would stick.

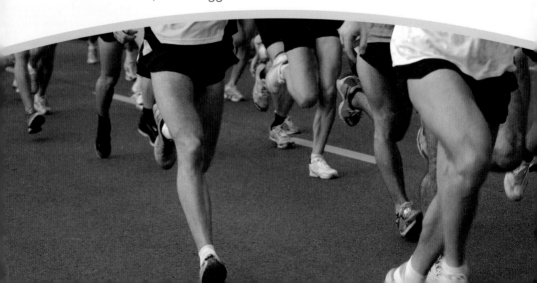

The point is that for many people what they need to be looking for as they begin their habit change journey is in fact *one ridiculously small step or goal.* That's all that is required. When habit change is hard, daunting, or discouraging, that first step needs to be not just small, but *ridiculously* small. Why? There are several important reasons:[70]

1. **It will be easier for you to imagine yourself doing it.**

2. **It will overcome your inner fear of change.**

3. **It will help conquer procrastination.**

4. **It will get you moving and overcome loads of built in inertia.**

5. **It will boost your self-confidence.**

6. **It will give you an early win, something to celebrate.**

7. **Once accomplished, it will motivate you to continue.**

In that light, the first tiny step is not ridiculous at all! When it comes to habit creation, small is a really big deal. You always want to keep vividly in mind the mental picture of the new habit being fully incorporated into your life. But as far as the process of getting there is concerned, *you only need to plan the next ridiculously small step and then, after accomplishing that, the next.* Somewhere down the road those steps can get larger.

One woman who knew she should exercise purchased an expensive treadmill for her home but could not bring herself to use it. Exercise remained an illusive, unsavory goal. Someone then introduced her to the wonders of small steps. For the first month, she just *stood* on the treadmill without walking as she sipped her coffee and read her newspaper. Over that time she began to associate the treadmill with her morning routine. During the following month, after finishing her coffee, she walked on the device for *one minute* each day, adding one minute each week. Slowly she developed a tolerance for exercise. Over time her "ridiculous" small steps grew into a firm habit of one mile a day![71]

The concept that small is big has a name in Japanese, *kaisen.* It is a strategy for change that utilizes tiny, continuous improvements. It was introduced to the island nation after World War II. It is based on the realization that change, even positive change, activates fear which is the basis of the well known flight or fight response. We get anxious and run, avoid or deny. The small steps in *kaisen* don't set off the fight or flight response, giving us a far better shot at success.[72]

For those who might get impatient, Dr. Robert Maurer comments, "If you find yourself growing frustrated with the pace of change, ask yourself: *Isn't slow change better than what I've experienced before… which is no change at all?*"[73]

In God's sight, small things can be very valuable. Jesus talked about a mustard seed, for instance.

> *"Another parable He put forth to them, saying: "The kingdom of heaven is like a mustard seed, which a man took and sowed in his field, which indeed is the least of all the seeds; but when it is grown it is greater than the herbs and becomes a tree, so that the birds of the air come and nest in its branches"* (Matthew 13:31-32, NKJV).

To the untrained eye, a mustard seed is not the most impressive seed on the store rack: 1/8th the size of a grain of rice;[74] 1/3 the size of a poppy seed.[75]

Calling the mustard seed the smallest of all seeds was a proverbial saying in Jesus' day. Amazingly, despite appearances, it can grow to the size of a tree from eight to twelve feet high.[76] Birds even nest there. Imagine a male bird, who's courting a female, pointing to a mustard seed on the ground and saying, "Honey, that thing is where we're going to build our home someday." Crazy? Not if you understand.

Applying the mustard seed parable to habit creation, our seemingly small steps have tremendous meaning and potential.

Christ also said that in order for growth to happen, the farmer has to first *take* the mustard seed and then *sow it.* In other words, we have to seize the opportunity and actively invest it in our own future. Jesus invites us to underwhelm ourselves with how tiny our first steps are and then see what can come of them as he infuses us with his power to grow.

Do you hate cleaning? Home organizing guru Marla Cilley invented what is called the "5-Minute Room Rescue." You set the oven timer for five minutes. Then go to the messiest room in the house and start cleaning – anything, any way. When the timer buzzes you stop, with a clear conscience and a certain measure of self-satisfaction. The next day you do the same.

What good is five minutes? It gets you going, which is the hardest part. And once you start and see the good result, you probably won't stay at five minutes very long. The authors of the book *Switch* comment, "You'll start to take pride in your accomplishments – starting with the clean sink, then the clean bathroom, then the clean downstairs area – and that pride and confidence will build on itself. A virtuous circle."[77]

*To be most helpful and effective, whatever small goal you choose needs to have certain characteristics.* It should be *specific and measurable,* which means you can tell when it is accomplished. Goals such as, "Becoming more kind," "Being more patient," and "Having more happiness" are far too imprecise to have any meaning. They are "fuzzy goals." Notice that they all usually contain the word "more." How can you take satisfaction in an attainment when you can't really know whether you've attained it or not?

Another key point in setting goals is to *avoid absolutes.* Saying things like, "I'll *never* eat fried cream puffs again," or "I'll *never* be late again," sets the bar far too high. We may never intend to do those things again, but we can only take one day at a time. "Never again" can be overwhelmingly scary. It can shut us down or set us up for deep discouragement when we fall short. The truth is that every day is a fresh start and new opportunity.

Once you've accomplished your first small step, take what you have learned from that experience and figure out the next little step, and after that the next, and so on. Repeat until you arrive at where you want to be.

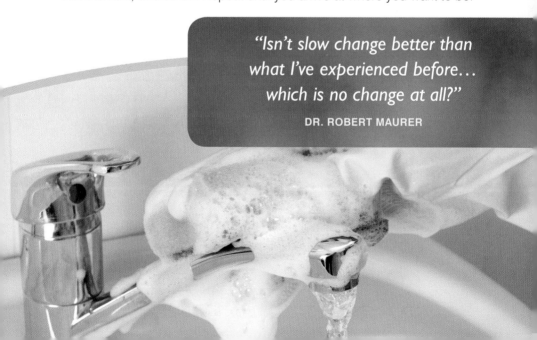

> *"Isn't slow change better than what I've experienced before... which is no change at all?"*
>
> **DR. ROBERT MAURER**

# YOUR ABUNDANT LIVING
# ACTION PLAN

Setting proper goals is an important part of what we might call your "Abundant Living Action Plan." Having such a plan is a major key to success. In order to increase the potential for victory in the creation of your new habit, it is best to incorporate the following elements into your plan:

1. **Write down the description of your new habit** that you developed in lesson 7 and the *initial small step* you anticipate implementing from the earlier part of this lesson. You can then record additional steps as you develop them. It is vital to break big goals into small, manageable steps and patiently take them one by one.

2. **Now make a firm commitment to ACT.** Resolve to make it happen. Make the choice and follow through. Get excited about the possibilities that lie ahead then start moving. Believe in yourself and move forward with confidence.

   *"One of the greatest allies of transformation is intention – the drive to do something different. Intention is not wanting, wishing, or hoping; it's the determination to do…With intention, we indicate to ourselves that we are going to do something no matter what."*[78]

3. **Set a date to start pursuing your initial goal** and tell someone about it. Tomorrow is a great time to begin. Don't wait too long and let your resolve begin to wane. Whatever date you set, telling someone about it makes it more real and provides accountability. Set dates for each of your subsequent goals as well.[79]

4. **Track your progress.** It will be especially helpful down the road to look back and see how all of your many little steps are starting to add up. Many people have found that some form of tracking was vital to their success.[80]

5. **Plan for times of failure.** All significant change involves periodically tripping up and falling flat on our face. It's completely normal. Plan on it ahead of time, expect it, and think of ways *now* to encourage yourself when it occurs. Learn from these stumbles. Think of them as positives because they mean you are stretching, making things happen. Try to find at least one person who can be your support system and help you avoid discouragement when you hit some speed bumps along the way.[81]

6. **Treat yourself kindly.** Reward yourself often and celebrate every little inch of progress. Especially celebrate whenever you refuse to let slip-ups become give-ups.

7. **Don't hesitate to call upon God's resources and aid.** The apostle Paul offers these words of encouragement, "Let us have confidence, then, and approach God's throne, where there is grace. There we will receive mercy and find grace to help us *just when we need it*" (Hebrews 4:16, GNT). The apostle also pens this wonderfully optimistic perspective on your future through God's assistance:

   *"Now to him who is able to do immeasurably more than all we ask or imagine, according to his power that is at work within us, to him be glory…for ever and ever!" (Ephesians 3:20-21, NIV).*

*Here are some examples of potential small first steps (we might call them Mustard Seed Steps):*

| Definition of New Habit | Potential Small First Steps |
|---|---|
| Have a bright, healthy smile. | Start developing a floss routine by flossing one tooth each day for a month. |
| Masters degree in hand, I begin my new career. | Do an Internet search of potential schools. |
| My family asking for "More veggies please." | Purchase a book on healthy cooking. |
| Rolling around on the floor with my kids as we laugh together. | Write "Family Time" into my appointment |
| Crossing the finish line in marathons. | Lay out my jogging clothes before going to bed. |
| I will treat myself the way I imagine Jesus treating me. | Write an affirming letter from God to myself and post it on a mirror. |

**Important Notice:** *The eight lessons you have just studied are Part 1 of the habit development series. You'll need the eight additional lessons in Part 2 to complete your Abundant Living journey and take it to the next level. Don't miss this opportunity to expand your understanding and give yourself the best possible chance for success!*

# DISCUSSION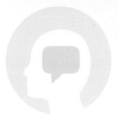

Have you ever been overwhelmed by the complexity and/or immensity of a task and felt like giving up? Give an example.

.............................................................................................

.............................................................................................

Do you have any personal experience with the power of small steps in your life?

.............................................................................................

.............................................................................................

If you have begun to define the new habit you want to pursue, what is the most ridiculously small step you can imagine taking to get started?

.............................................................................................

.............................................................................................

Which of the following is a "fuzzy goal"? Why?
- ○ Purchase 1 percent fat milk when I shop for groceries.
- ○ Take a cold shower once a week.
- ○ Become a better neighbor.
- ○ Read one chapter from the Bible each day.

.............................................................................................

.............................................................................................

What task have you successfully completed in the past? What clues does that give you regarding your ability to persist in habit creation?

.............................................................................................

.............................................................................................

If you have started the habit change journey during this lesson series, what have been some of your challenges and successes?

.............................................................................................

.............................................................................................

How would you track your progress with your new habit?

.............................................................................................

.............................................................................................

Where do you find encouragement to help you deal with some failure?

.............................................................................................

.............................................................................................

# SHARING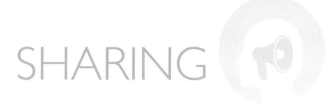

## OPPORTUNITY #8:

- Pray as a group for God to open the way for you to share something from these lessons to help someone else.

- Keep your radar up each day for opportunities.

**How this lesson can impact our Choices and Outlook**

CHOICE:

1. Change is a series of continuous small choices.

2. Our choices as we move forward with habit creation should be based on an "Abundant Living Action Plan."

OUTLOOK:

1. Small, tiny steps help develop and maintain an attitude of hope.

2. We should take pride and satisfaction in each step forward, no matter how insignificant it may appear.

## ABUNDANT LIVING THOUGHT

A goal should be specific and measurable, which means you can tell when it is accomplished. Goals such as, "Becoming more kind," "Being more patient," and "Having more happiness" are far too imprecise to have any meaning.

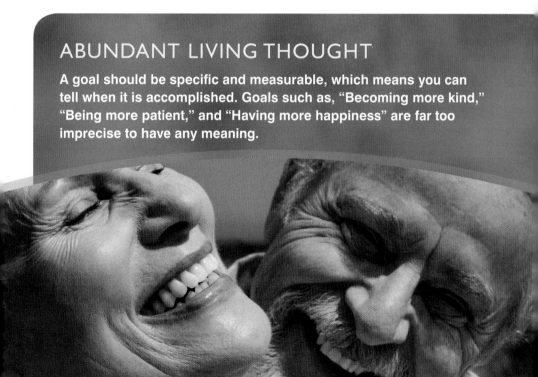

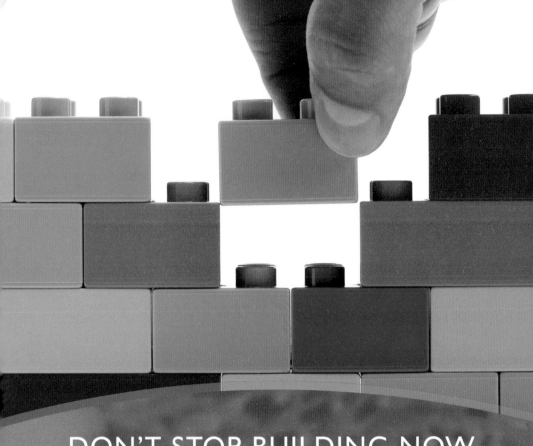

# DON'T STOP BUILDING NOW
## FILL IN THE MISSING PIECES

You already have a number of key building blocks in place from what you learned in Part 1 of "Creating Healthy Habits for Life." To get the rest of the pieces be sure to pick up part 2. It is Guide #7 in the CREATION Health Life Guide Series.

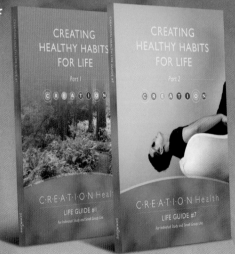

PARTS 1&2: **CHOICE & OUTLOOK**

# ABOUT THE AUTHOR

Kim Johnson is a popular writer, speaker, and fervent advocate for holistic living. As the author of three books, eleven lesson series, and many articles, his writings focus on healthy living and spiritual connectedness. His materials have been used in hundreds of churches throughout North America and internationally as well.

Johnson is an ordained minister with more than 35 years of experience as a parish pastor and church administrator. Over the years, his work with parishioners emphasized principles of whole-person health as a path to optimum mental, physical, social, and spiritual well-being. His later work with pastors and church leaders emphasized skill development such as vision casting, goal setting, support systems, relationship management, and accountability. Johnson has put his experience of working with pastors and parishioners to use in the CREATION Health Life Guide Series by creating a resource ideally suited for use in churches, small groups or individual study.

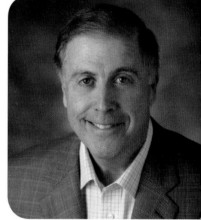

Johnson holds a Master of Divinity degree and received his Bachelor of Arts in theology. He currently serves as Director of Resource Development for churches in the state of Florida. His personal interests include reading, classical music, art and book festivals, kayaking, traveling, volunteering, and small group study. He and his wife Ann make their home in Orlando.

**Author Acknowledgements:** It has been a great privilege for me to be associated with the team of dedicated individuals who helped in various ways to make these CREATION Health Life Guides available. I would like to single out my wife Ann and daughter Stefanie, whose feedback and suggestions were always characterized by unfailing support and clear-eyed honesty. I have also received invaluable guidance and encouragement from Mike Cauley, Tim Nichols, Nick Howard, and Jim Epperson. Finally, I want to thank the group of local pastors who met with me personally and provided a wonderful forum for evaluating the lesson drafts.

# NOTES

1.  Garry Poole, *The Complete Book of Questions* (Grand Rapids, MI: Zondervan, 2003), 21.

2.  Garry Poole, *The Complete Book of Questions,* 59.

3.  Garry Poole, *The Complete Book of Questions,* 80.

4.  Garry Poole, *The Complete Book of Questions,* 73.

5.  James Claiborn and Cherry Pedrick, *The Habit Change Workbook* (Oakland, CA: New Harbinger Publications, Inc., 2001), 158.

6.  Des Cummings and Monica Reed, *CREATION Health Discovery* (Orlando, FL: Florida Hospital Publishing, 2005), 77.

7.  John Maxwell, *Attitude 101* (Nashville, TN: Thomas Nelson, 2003), 15.

8.  Garry Poole, *The Complete Book of Questions* (Grand Rapids, MI: Zondervan, 2003), 117.

9.  Garry Poole, *The Complete Book of Questions,* 66.

10. Sonja Lyubomirsky, *The How of Happiness* (New York, NY: The Penguin Press, 2007), 53-55.

11. Sonja Lyubomirsky, *The How of Happiness,* 55-56.

12. Claudia Wallis, "The New Science of Happiness," *Time,* January 17, 2005, http://www.authentichappiness.sas.upenn.edu/images/timemagazine/Time-Happiness.pdf.

13. Sonya Lyubomirsky, *The How of Happiness,* 21.

14. Sonya Lyubomirsky, *The How of Happiness,* 39.

15. Claudia Wallis, "The New Science of Happiness." *Time,* January 17, 2005, http://www.authentichappiness.sas.upenn.edu/images/timemagazine/Time-Happiness.pdf.

16. Robert A. Emmons, *Thanks* (Boston, MA: Houghton Mifflin Company, 2007), 6.

17. Sonya Lyubomirsky, *The How of Happiness,* 99-100.

18. Debbie Macomber, *One Simple Act*, (New York, NY: Howard Books, 2009), 14.

19. Debbie Macomber, *One Simple Act,* 15-16.

20. Claudia Wallis, "The New Science of Happiness." *Time,* January 17, 2005, http://www.authentichappiness.sas.upenn.edu/images/timemagazine/Time-Happiness.pdf; Sonya Lyubomirsky, *The How of Happiness,* 95-100.

21. "The Benefits of Gratitude," *motivateus.com,* January 23, 2009, http://www.motivateus.com/stories/gratitude.htm.

22. Meladee McCarty and Hanoch McCarty, *Acts of Kindness* (Deerfield Beach, FL: Health Communications, Inc.,1994), 5.

23. Debbie Macomber, *One Simple Act,* 20-23.

24. Leon Morris, *The Gospel of According to Matthew* (Grand Rapids, MI: William B. Eerdmans Publishing Co., 1992), 378.

25. David Kilgour, "The Power of Generosity to Promote Transformation," November 13, 2005, http://www.david-kilgour.com/mp/Generosity.htm.

26. Dave Toycen, *The Power of Generosity* (Ontario, Canada: Harper Collins Publishers Ltd., 2004), 14.

27. Sonya Lyubomirsky, *The How of Happiness,* 192.

28. Sonya Lyubomirsky, *The How of Happiness,* 193-199.

29. Sonya Lyubomirsky, *The How of Happiness,* 181.

30. Sonya Lyubomirsky, *The How of Happiness,* 251.

31. Garry Poole, *The Complete Book of Questions* (Grand Rapids, MI: Zondervan, 2003), 49.

32. "How to Apply Jeremiah 29 (understand Jeremiah 29:11-13)." eHow, at: http://www.ehow.com/how_5473475_apply-jeremiah-understand-jeremiah.html. Accessed 07/03/12.

33. Gretchen Rubin, *The Happiness Project* (New York, NY: Harper Collins Publishers, 2011), 259.

34. Charles and Frances Hunter, *Healing Through Humor* (Lake Mary, FL: Creation House Press, 2003), xi.

35. Michelle W. Murray, "Laughter Is the Best Medicine," July 14, 2009, http://www.umm.edu/features/laughter.htm.

36. Gretchen Rubin, *The Happiness Project,* 261.

37. Elisha Goldstein, PhD, The Joy of Play, *AOL Healthy Living,* June 16, 2011, http://www.huffingtonpost.com/elisha-goldstein-phd/joy-of-play_b_876993.html

38. Elilsha Goldstein, PhD, *The Joy of Play.*

39. Stephen R. Covey, *The 7 Habits of Highly Effective People* (New York, NY: Simon and Schuster, 1989), 55.

40. Cari LaGrange Murphy, *Create Change Now* (Mustang, Oklahoma: Tate Publishing & Enterprises, LLC., 2009), 102.

41. Adapted from Laura Whitworth, Karen Kimsey-House, Henry Kimsey-House, Phillip Sandahl, *Co-Active Coaching* (Boston, MA: Davies-Black, 2007), 135.

42. Garry Poole, *The Complete Book of Questions* (Grand Rapids, MI: Zondervan, 2003), 65.

43. Garry Poole, *The Complete Book of Questions,* 118.

44. *The American Heritage Dictionary* (Boston, MA: Houghton Mifflin Company, 1976), 586.

45. William Barclay, *The Gospel of Luke,* (Philadelphia, PA: The Westminster Press, 1975), 150.

46. Nannette Richford, "How Long Does a Butterfly Stay in a Chrysalis Cocoon?," http://www.ehow.com/about_4572522_does-butterfly-stay-chrysalis-cocoon.html.

47. Hal Urban, *Choices That Change Lives,* (New York, NY: Simon & Schuster, 2006), xxii.

48. Hal Urban, *Choices That Change Lives,* 225.

49. *The American Heritage Dictionary,* 882.

50. John Maxwell, *Attitude 101* (Nashville, TN: Thomas Nelson, 2003), 22.

51. John Maxwell, *Attitude 101,* 43-44.

52. M.J. Ryan, *This Year I Will* (New York, NY: Broadway Books, 2006), 82.

53. Garry Poole, *The Complete Book of Questions* (Grand Rapids, MI: Zondervan, 2003), 119.

54. Garry Poole, *The Complete Book of Questions,* 41.

55. James O. Prochaska, John C. Norcross, Carlo C. DiClemente, *Changing for Good* (New York, NY: Harper Collins Publishers, 2006).

56. James O. Prochaska, John C. Norcross, Carlo C. DiClemente, *Changing for Good,* 79, 80, 96-97.

57. James O. Prochaska, John C. Norcross, Carlo C. DiClemente, *Changing for Good,* 125-126.

58. James O. Prochaska, John C. Norcross, Carlo C. DiClemente, *Changing for Good,* 146, 151, 157-158.

59. James O. Prochaska, John C. Norcross, Carlo C. DiClemente, *Changing for Good,* 176-194.

60. M.J. Ryan, *This Year I Will* (New York, NY: Broadway Books, 2006), 131-133.

61. M.J. Ryan, *This Year I Will,* 132.

62. M.J. Ryan, *This Year I Will,* 72.

63. Hyrum W. Smith, *What Matters Most* (New York, NY: Franklin Covey Co., 2000), 83.

64. Hyrum W. Smith, *What Matters Most,* 91- 92.

65. M.J. Ryan, *This Year I Will,* 155.

66. M.J. Ryan, *This Year I Will,* 43.

67. M.J. Ryan, *This Year I Will,* 53-55.

68. M.J. Ryan, *This Year I Will,* 28.

69. Garry Poole, *The Complete Book of Questions* (Grand Rapids, MI: Zondervan, 2003), 35.

70. M.J. Ryan, *This Year I Will* (New York, NY: Broadway Books, 2006), 77-78.

71. Robert Maurer, *One Small Step Can Change Your Life* (New York, NY: Workman Publishing, 2004), 100.

72. M.J. Ryan, *This Year I Will,* 77-78.

73. Robert Maurer, *One Small Step Can Change Your Life,* 101.

74. Maurice Burke, "How Big Is a Mustard Seed," *Gospel Globe,* July 21, 2010, http://www.gospelglobe.com/Opinion/how-big-is-a-mustard-seed/index.php.

75. David, "How Big Is a Mustard Seed," *The I-61 Project Blog,* May 16, 2009, http://i61project.blogspot.com/2009/05/how-big-is-mustard-seed.html.

76. Leon Morris, *The Gospel According to Matthew* (Grand Rapids, MI: William B. Eerdmans Publishing Company, 1992), 652.

77. Chip Heath and Dan Heath, *Switch* (New York, NY: Broadway Books, 2010), 130-131.

78. M.J. Ryan, *This Year I Will,* 88-89.

79. James O. Prochaska, John C. Norcross, Carlo C. Diclemente, *Changing for Good* (New York, NY: HarperCollins, 2006), 155.

80. M.J. Ryan, *This Year I Will,* 100.

81. M.J. Ryan, *This Year I Will,* 101, 193; James O. Prochaska, John C. Norcross, Carlo C. Diclement, *Changing for Good,* 158,

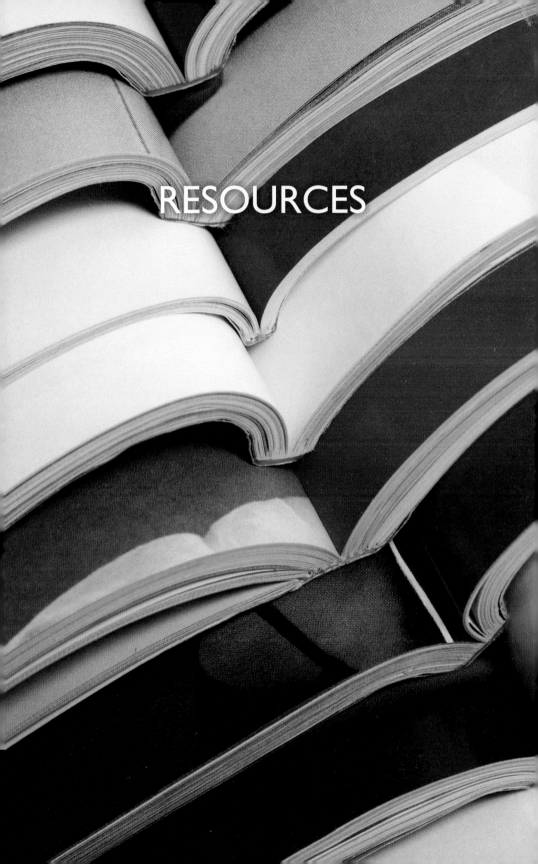
RESOURCES

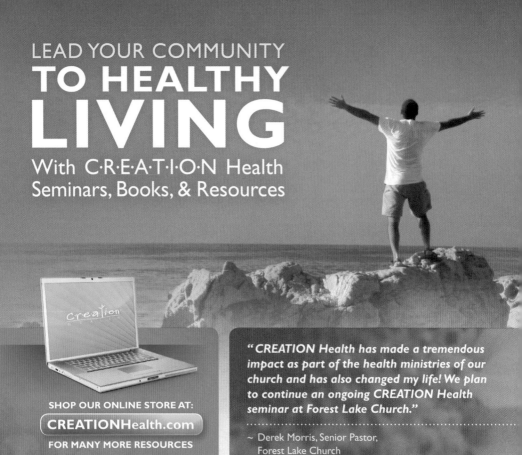

# LEAD YOUR COMMUNITY
# TO HEALTHY
# LIVING

## With C·R·E·A·T·I·O·N Health
## Seminars, Books, & Resources

SHOP OUR ONLINE STORE AT:

**CREATIONHealth.com**

FOR MANY MORE RESOURCES

*"CREATION Health has made a tremendous impact as part of the health ministries of our church and has also changed my life! We plan to continue an ongoing CREATION Health seminar at Forest Lake Church."*

~ Derek Morris, Senior Pastor,
Forest Lake Church

## SEMINAR MATERIALS

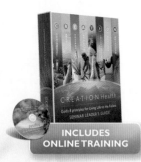

INCLUDES
ONLINE TRAINING

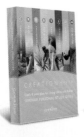

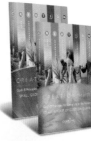

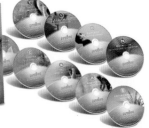

### Leader Guide

Everything a leader needs to conduct this seminar successfully, including key questions to facilitate group discussion and PowerPoint™ presentations for each of the eight principles.

### Participant Guide

A study guide with essential information from each of the eight lessons along with outlines, self assessments, and questions for people to fill-in as they follow along.

### Small Group Kit

It's easy to lead a small group using the CREATION Health videos, the Small Group Leaders Guide and the Small Group Discussion Guide.

## GUIDES AND ASSESSMENTS

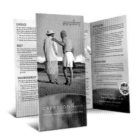
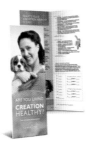
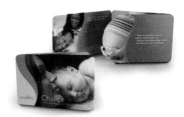

### Senior Guide

Share the CREATION Health principles with seniors and help them be healthier and happier as they live life to the fullest.

### Self-Assessment

This instrument raises awareness about how CREATION Healthy a person is in each of the eight major areas of wellness.

### Pregnancy Guides

Expert advice on how to be CREATION Healthy while expecting.

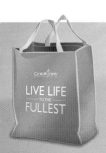

### GET ORGANIZED!

### Tote Bag

A convenient way for bringing CREATION Health materials to and from class.

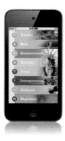

### Smartphone App

The free CREATION Health App supplies daily health tips, weekly CREATION Conversation videos, and refreshing virtual vacations to break away from your day.

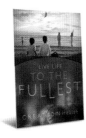

### Presentation Folder

Keep CREATION Health notes and resources organized and in one place.

### Pocket Guide

A tool for keeping people committed to living all of the CREATION Health principles daily.

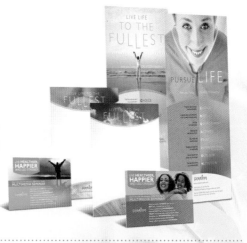

## MARKETING MATERIALS

### Postcards, Posters, Stationary, and more

You can effectively advertise and generate community excitement about your CREATION Health seminar with a wide range of available marketing materials such as enticing postcards, flyers, posters, and more.

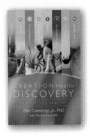

### CREATION Health Discovery (Softcover)

*CREATION Health Discovery* takes the 8 essential principles of CREATION Health and melds them together to form the blueprint for the health we yearn for and the life we are intended to live.

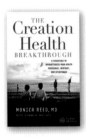

### CREATION Health Breakthrough (Hardcover)

Blending science and lifestyle recommendations, Monica Reed, MD, prescribes eight essentials that will help reverse harmful health habits and prevent disease. Discover how intentional choices, rest, environment, activity, trust, relationships, outlook, and nutrition can put a person on the road to wellness. Features a three-day total body rejuvenation therapy and four-phase life transformation plan.

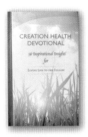

### CREATION Health Devotional (English: Hardcover / Spanish: Softcover)

Stories change lives. Stories can inspire health and healing. In this devotional you will discover stories about experiencing God's grace in the tough times, God's delight in triumphant times, and God's presence in peaceful times. Based on the eight timeless principles of wellness: Choice, Rest, Environment, Activity, Trust, Interpersonal relationships, Outlook, Nutrition.

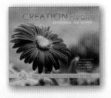

### CREATION Health Devotional for Women (English)

Written for women by women, the *CREATION Health Devotional for Women* is based on the principles of whole-person wellness represented in CREATION Health. Spirits will be lifted and lives rejuvenated by the message of each unique chapter. This book is ideal for women's prayer groups, to give as a gift, or just to buy for your own edification and encouragement.

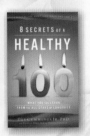

### 8 Secrets of a Healthy 100 (Softcover)

Can you imagine living to a Healthy 100 years of age? Dr. Des Cummings Jr., explores the principles practiced by the All-stars of Longevity to live longer and more abundantly. Take a journey through the 8 Secrets and you will be inspired to imagine living to a Healthy 100.

### Forgive To Live (English: Hardcover / Spanish: Softcover)

*In Forgive to Live* Dr. Tibbits presents the scientifically proven steps for forgiveness – taken from the first clinical study of its kind conducted by Stanford University and Florida Hospital.

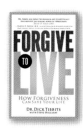

### Forgive To Live Workbook (Softcover)

This interactive guide will show you how to forgive – insight by insight, step by step – in a workable plan that can effectively reduce your anger, improve your health, and put you in charge of your life again, no matter how deep your hurts.

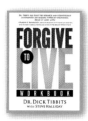

### Forgive To Live Devotional (Hardcover)

In his powerful new devotional Dr. Dick Tibbits reveals the secret to forgiveness. This compassionate devotional is a stirring look at the true meaning of forgiveness. Each of the 56 spiritual insights includes motivational Scripture, an inspirational prayer, and two thought-provoking questions. The insights are designed to encourage your journey as you begin to *Forgive to Live*.

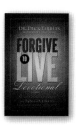

### Forgive To Live God's Way (Softcover)

Forgiveness is so important that our very lives depend on it. Churches teach us that we should forgive, but how do you actually learn to forgive? In this spiritual workbook noted author, psychologist, and ordained minister Dr. Dick Tibbits takes you step-by-step through an eight-week forgiveness format that is easy to understand and follow.

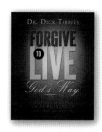

### Forgive To Live Leader's Guide

Perfect for your community, church, small group or other settings.

**The Forgive to Live Leader's Guide Includes:**

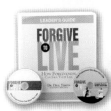

- 8 Weeks of pre-designed PowerPoint™ presentations.
- Professionally designed customizable marketing materials and group handouts on CD-Rom.
- Training directly from author of Forgive to Live Dr. Dick Tibbits across 6 audio CDs.
- Media coverage DVD.
- CD-Rom containing all files in digital format for easy home or professional printing.
- A copy of the first study of its kind conducted by Stanford University and Florida Hospital showing a link between decreased blood pressure and forgiveness.

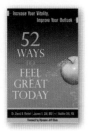

## 52 Ways to Feel Great Today (Softcover)

Wouldn't you love to feel great today? Changing your outlook and injecting energy into your day often begins with small steps. In *52 Ways to Feel Great Today*, you'll discover an abundance of simple, inexpensive, fun things you can do to make a big difference in how you feel today and every day. Tight on time? No problem. Each chapter is written as a short, easy-to-implement idea. Every idea is supported by at least one true story showing how helpful implementing the idea has proven to someone a lot like you. The stories are also included to encourage you to be as inventive, imaginative, playful, creative, or adventuresome as you can.

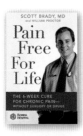

## Pain Free For Life (Hardcover)

In *Pain Free For Life*, Scott C. Brady, MD, – founder of Florida Hospital's Brady Institute for Health – shares for the first time with the general public his dramatically successful solution for chronic back pain, Fibromyalgia, chronic headaches, Irritable bowel syndrome and other "impossible to cure" pains. Dr. Brady leads pain-racked readers to a pain-free life using powerful mind-body-spirit strategies used at the Brady Institute – where more than 80 percent of his chronic-pain patients have achieved 80-100 percent pain relief within weeks.

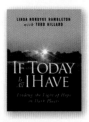

## If Today Is All I Have (Softcover)

At its heart, Linda's captivating account chronicles the struggle to reconcile her three dreams of experiencing life as a "normal woman" with the tough realities of her medical condition. Her journey is punctuated with insights that are at times humorous, painful, provocative, and life-affirming.

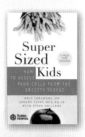

## SuperSized Kids (Hardcover)

In *SuperSized Kids*, Walt Larimore, MD, and Sherri Flynt, MPH, RD, LD, show how the mushrooming childhood obesity epidemic is destroying children's lives, draining family resources, and pushing America dangerously close to a total healthcare collapse – while also explaining, step by step, how parents can work to avert the coming crisis by taking control of the weight challenges facing every member of their family.

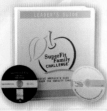

## SuperFit Family Challenge – Leader's Guide

Perfect for your community, church, small group or other settings.
**The SuperFit Family Challenge Leader's Guide Includes:**

- 8 Weeks of pre-designed PowerPoint™ presentations.
- Professionally designed marketing materials and group handouts from direct mailers to reading guides.
- Training directly from Author Sherri Flynt, MPH, RD, LD, across 6 audio CDs.
- Media coverage and FAQ on DVD.

# LIVE YOUR LIFE
# TO THE FULLEST

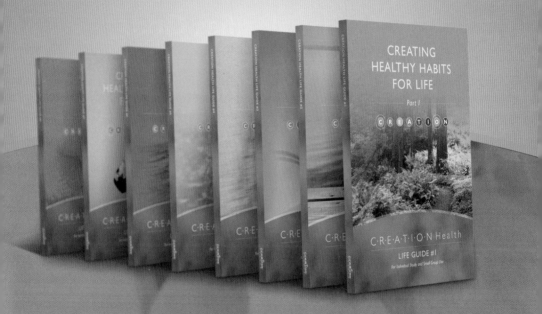

# C·R·E·A·T·I·O·N Health

## LIFE GUIDE SERIES

8 Guides. 8 Principles. One Powerful Message.
Packed with fresh insights on abundant living.
For Individual Study and Small Group Use.

Perfect for churches, schools, universities, and faith-based businesses.

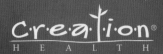

# YOUR PATH TO A HEALTHY 100

**(C) CHOICE** – First we make choices—then choices make us. To gain optimum value in life you first need to choose a destination. Next, learn the success steps for creating habits that will lead you to a healthy destiny.

**(R) REST** – Rest is powerful. It refreshes, rejuvenates, and rebuilds the mind, body, and spirit. Rest empowers you to function at your best. Optimally, rest includes a good night's sleep and time to unwind daily, weekly, and annually.

**(E) ENVIRONMENT** – Environment is what lies outside our bodies yet affects what takes place inside us. All of our senses—sight, smell, sound, touch, and taste—can influence our health, either positively or negatively.

**(A) ACTIVITY** – Activity includes both mental and physical movement and development. The mind and the body are intimately connected. A fit mind promotes a healthy body, and a healthy body promotes a fit mind.

**(T) TRUST** – Trust in God speaks to the important relationship between spirituality and healing. Research shows that our faith, beliefs, and hopes can play an important role in our health. It may even help us live longer.

**(I) INTERPERSONAL** – Interpersonal Relationships are vital to your well-being. Knowing you have the love and support of others can contribute to improved health, while toxic relationships can lead to negative health results.

**(O) OUTLOOK** – Recent research suggests that your attitude powerfully influences your health. Having a positive outlook not only colors your perspective on life, it is one of the best gifts you can give yourself.

**(N) NUTRITION** – Food is the fuel that drives your life. It can rev you up or slow you down. Take time to evaluate your intake. Even small improvements, done regularly, can supercharge your health. Eat for energy. Eat for life!

For other life changing
resources, visit us at:
CREATIONHealth.com

12.99

9 780983 988113
ISBN 978-0-9839881-1-3

51299